Bringing Art to Life

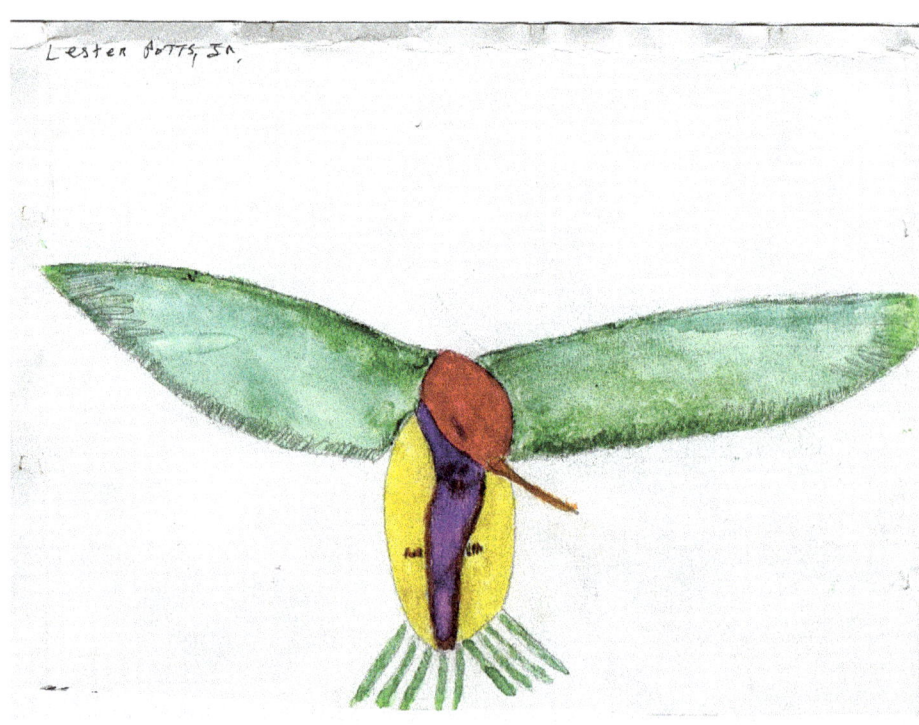

Bringing Art to Life

Reflections on Dementia and the
Transforming Power of Art and Relationships

Daniel C. Potts

Foreword by Emily Broman Phelps

RESOURCE *Publications* · Eugene, Oregon

BRINGING ART TO LIFE
Reflections on Dementia and the Transforming Power of Art and Relationships

Copyright © 2022 Daniel C. Potts. All rights reserved. Except for brief quotations in critical publications or reviews, no part of this book may be reproduced in any manner without prior written permission from the publisher. Write: Permissions, Wipf and Stock Publishers, 199 W. 8th Ave., Suite 3, Eugene, OR 97401.

Resource Publications
An Imprint of Wipf and Stock Publishers
199 W. 8th Ave., Suite 3
Eugene, OR 97401

www.wipfandstock.com

PAPERBACK ISBN: 978-1-6667-3696-0
HARDCOVER ISBN: 978-1-6667-9591-2
EBOOK ISBN: 978-1-6667-9592-9

06/28/22

Daniel C. Potts holds the copyright for all the art, photographs, and poetry contained in this book.

Scripture quotations from The Authorized (King James) Version. Rights in the Authorized Version in the United Kingdom are vested in the Crown. Reproduced by permission of the Crown's patentee, Cambridge University Press.

This book is dedicated in memory of the Reverend Dr. Richard L. Morgan, pastor, pioneer in the field of spirituality and aging, mentor, author, activist, champion, and humble man of faith, without whose encouragement and guidance the book would not have come to fruition.

Additionally, this book is dedicated to my wife, Ellen W. Potts, MBA, without whose unconditional love, support, and encouragement I would have little to write about, and with whom I will gratefully continue to partner in advocacy and in life.

Finally, this book is dedicated to all past, current, and future participants in the Bringing Art to Life program from Cognitive Dynamics Foundation, including persons living with dementia, students, art therapists, musicians, other artists and guest faculty, researchers, care partners, collaborators, and financial supporters, as well as those who have inspired any truth contained herein.

Creativity is seen as leading to well-being by helping us articulate a story about who we are (coherence), exercise a purpose, and demonstrating the significance or value of our lives . . . Creativity can also help us build a legacy, something that can live beyond us and that can reduce the stress, anxiety, or at the very least the unsettledness we can feel when we face mortality.

—ANNE BASTING[1]

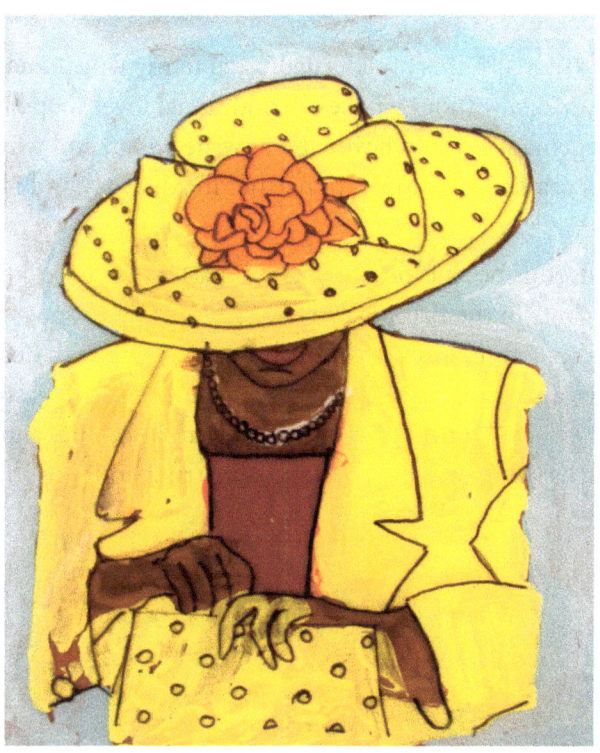

1. Basting, *Creative Care*, 46.

Contents

Foreword by Emily Broman Phelps | xi
Acknowledgements | xv
Illustrations | xvii

Part I: Prelude and Program Description

Prelude | 3
BATL Program Description | 13
Building a Culture of Compassion | 18
The Room | 25
Thoughts on the Spiritual in Dementia Care | 29

Part II: The Stories

A Word about the Stories | 37

Maria and Madre | 39
A Day Like Today | 43
Helping Miss Carrie | 47
Ernie's Hands | 50
A Smile and a Handshake | 54
He Taught Us How to Listen | 58
Some Things Are Meant to Be | 61
Beyond the Blue | 67
Art with Mary | 72
Amazing Grace with Aretha | 76
Miss Lola's Purse | 79
Keep Going! | 82

Part III: Poetry Inspired by BATL

Thoughts on Writing Poetry | 89

A Face | 91
A Heart That Knows Your Name | 92
A Love-Washed Healing | 93
An Elder's Hope | 95
Bringing Art to Life | 96
Come On, Join the Choir | 97
Do You Hear Me? | 98
Hey, Do I Know You? | 99
Hands upon My Window | 100
He Can't | 101
Hunter County | 102
I'll Remember What I Named You | 103
Life Lesson | 104
Love Holds Us | 105
Message in a Bottle | 106
Poem for an Elder | 107
Somebody | 109
Someone Is There | 110
Someone to Guide Me | 111
Story Time with Old Folks | 112
Take Me to Your Hiding Place | 113
The Third Friday in October | 114
This Is Home | 115
Those Girls Came to Visit | 116
Was That You? | 117
What Are You Planning to Paint? | 119
When You're Lost | 120
Where the Forest Meets the Sky | 122
Wherever She May Go | 123
Yesterday | 124
You Asked Me if I Remember | 125
You Chose to Listen | 127
You—Me | 129

Part IV: Lessons Learned
　Pillars of Personhood | 133
　A Paradigm Honoring Selfhood & Relationships in Dementia Care | 133
　Thirty-One Lessons | 135

Part V: Final Thoughts
　Showing Me Back to Me | 141
　Postlude | 145

About the Author | 149
Bibliography | 151

Foreword

I COULD TELL YOU exactly what I was doing on that first day. When I first learned about Bringing Art to Life (BATL).

My good friend Michael had tracked me down in the Student Government Association office at the University of Alabama. I was sitting at a communal table doing office hours, positioned with a strategic view of the clock and the doorway. He invited me to an interest meeting—something about painting? "Do you really think I can leave? I'm supposed to be manning this desk." We both looked side to side at the emptiness of the office. That was enough for me to pack up and see what this painting class was all about. I mean, what was I really doing?

It was a fateful day. More than I could possibly express to the readers of this book. But perhaps what you will notice in the pages to come is a profound commitment to the depth of the human experience.

Over the past decade, Bringing Art to Life has engaged students with community-dwelling persons living with Alzheimer's disease and related dementias through art therapy and life-story preservation. To date, the initiative has expanded from Perry County, Alabama, to Tuscaloosa, Birmingham, and here in Chicago. Dr. Daniel Potts has worked with many dozens of students, countless family members, and many memorable persons with dementia to extend dignifying care that amplifies patient stories otherwise silenced by memory loss.

When I first started taking BATL, I was paired with Ms. Cora. At this point in my life, I had very little understanding of dementia. I also felt quite uncomfortable disclosing how little I could engage in the world of art. But I had registered for a process I expected to take about twelve weeks—we would spend some time with an intentionally chosen family, paint alongside an experienced art therapist, and compile life stories into an amalgam of sorts. Isn't that what we were really doing?

My classmate Jacqueline and I would drive fifty-seven miles into Alabama's countryside to Ms. Cora's house. Often, her son would greet us at the door, and we would set up a card table in the living room. Based on what we had already learned about Alzheimer's disease, I was rather surprised by Ms. Cora's ability to answer our questions and tell us stories. When we were painting or chatting, there wasn't anything she couldn't talk about. Jacqueline and I learned a wealth of stories about her teaching days, her Spanish class, and the chemistry teacher down the hall who gifted her exclusively yellow roses and became the love of her life.

It wasn't until we began compiling pieces for our life-story projects—the aforementioned amalgams—that we realized some details were fuzzy. We didn't have years or dates or chronicity in our project. And we concluded that filming a traditional interview or sewing a cohesive timeline would be much more difficult. Persons with dementia often have difficulty recognizing themselves on tape, in the mirror, or in the energy of their interactions with family. Numbers, facts, and specifics are a challenge for a tangled brain. The weight of perceptual disturbances, communication difficulties, and responsibilities of caregiving finally came into view. And then it dawned on me. What we were really doing.

This was my introduction to person-centered care and narrative impact. It drastically altered my mental framework of human communication. In BATL, eliciting life stories brought countercultural patience, emotional nuance, and multigenerational connectedness. The details, the flow, the timeline all were of little importance. The critical elements of our partnerships were the investment of time, the minutes spent in stories, and the reciprocation of those stories to amplify their impact.

On an otherwise overwhelming campus, BATL convened this curious crew of learners—artists, dancers, social workers, filmmakers, nurses, journalists, researchers, and aspiring doctors. Many of us had personal reasons we took this class—our "why." And this class built a bridge into the intimate lives of families surviving something similar. This is where I met the most admirable people I will ever meet, with an insatiable thirst for truth, equity, and connectedness.

It's been ten years.

In that decade, I've committed my professional and personal life to extending personhood into medicine and working with older adults where

Foreword

dignity in memory loss is severely lacking. It's been a meandering decade—as decades tend to be. But because of Bringing Art to Life, I've made my peace with the scenic route. And in a pattern of reflectiveness for which I thank dozens of families over the years, I trace my decision to pursue this path back to learning the inherent value in our stories.

In the most formative moments of my life, I never doubted the care and intention of Dr. Potts to carry us through our self-doubt into self-discovery, just as he does with persons with dementia. To adequately describe his mentorship during the following years would be impossible, but he continues to set my standard of intellect, compassion, and patient centeredness.

Herein are his stories—the essence of our being, the richness of personhood, and the art of human connectedness.

Emily Broman Phelps, MS, MD
Rush Medical College Class of 2021
Chicago, Illinois

Acknowledgements

GRATITUDE IS EXPRESSED TO the board of directors of the Cognitive Dynamics Foundation; executive arts director Angel Duncan (BATL cofounder and faculty); student facilitators Meg McCrummen Fowler, Dr. Emily Broman Phelps, Jacquelynn Myrick Dunn, Maggie Holmes, Zoe Berndt, Amanda Narkis, and Andrew Oreshkov; art therapists Sara Margaret Wade, Karen Gibbons, Amy Brown, Dr. Carrie Ezelle, Dr. Mildred Dawson-Hardy, Ally DeSantis, and Meredith Schroeder; and Art to Life Outreach facilitators Abby Holland, Madelyn Woo, and Morgan Roberts.

Thanks to Alabama Research Institute on Aging researchers Dr. Rebecca Allen (faculty), Dr. Keisha Carden, Candice Reel, and Dr. Anne Halli-Tierney (faculty); Dr. Rachel Raimist, Lynda Everman, Beth Sanders, and her team from LifeBio.com; Berna Huebner, Judy Holstein, the Reverend Dr. Cynthia Huling Hummel, and Brian LeBlanc; honorary faculty Naomi Feil, Dr. James M. Houston, the Reverend Dr. Richard Morgan, and Cathie Borrie; musicians Dr. Don Wendorf, Dr. Drexel Rayford, the Reverend Dr. Gary Furr, Melanie Rogers, Beth and Jeff Reinert, and Shades Mountain Air; funders The Alzheimer's Foundation of America, Dementia-Friendly Alabama; and others.

I would also like to thank the staff of the West Alabama Area Agency on Aging who administer The Virtual Dementia Tour© for our students; Carrie Shaw, Erin Washington, and their team at Embodied Labs; BATL-Chicago lead faculty Dr. Neelum Aggarwal, BATL-Chicago founding facilitators Dr. Angela Ray and Dr. Cyrus Alavi; BATL-Birmingham lead faculty Dr. Jessica Allen; directors and staff of McCoy Adult Dementia Daycare; Susanna Whitsett and staff at Founders Place Respite; Vicki Kerr, LaDerrick Smith, and the staff of Caring Days; Dad's late art teacher, George

Acknowledgements

Parker; Bill Lowe, Ann Brennon, and the staff, residents, and caregivers at Chicago Methodist Senior Services; pastors, staff, and congregants of First Presbyterian Church of Tuscaloosa; videographers Shelby Hadden, Greg Kubick, Lauren Musgrove, and Brian Covert; documentary producer and director Judith Murray; Dr. Jacqueline Morgan, Dr. Shane Sharp, and faculty and staff of the University of Alabama Honors College; proofreaders/editors Ellen Potts, Lynda Everman, and Dr. Don Wendorf; and my mother, Ethelda Potts.

Illustrations

THE TITLE PAGE CONTAINS the first painting of Lester E. Potts, Jr., an artist who had Alzheimer's disease (figure 1). With the exception of figure 4 (the mosaic at Caring Days in Tuscaloosa, Alabama), figure 7 (a participant in Bringing Art to Life and her students), and figure 8 (Lester and Daniel Potts) all other illustrations and photographs were created by persons living with cognitive impairment who participated in the Bringing Art to Life program from Cognitive Dynamics Foundation.

Part I

Prelude and Program Description

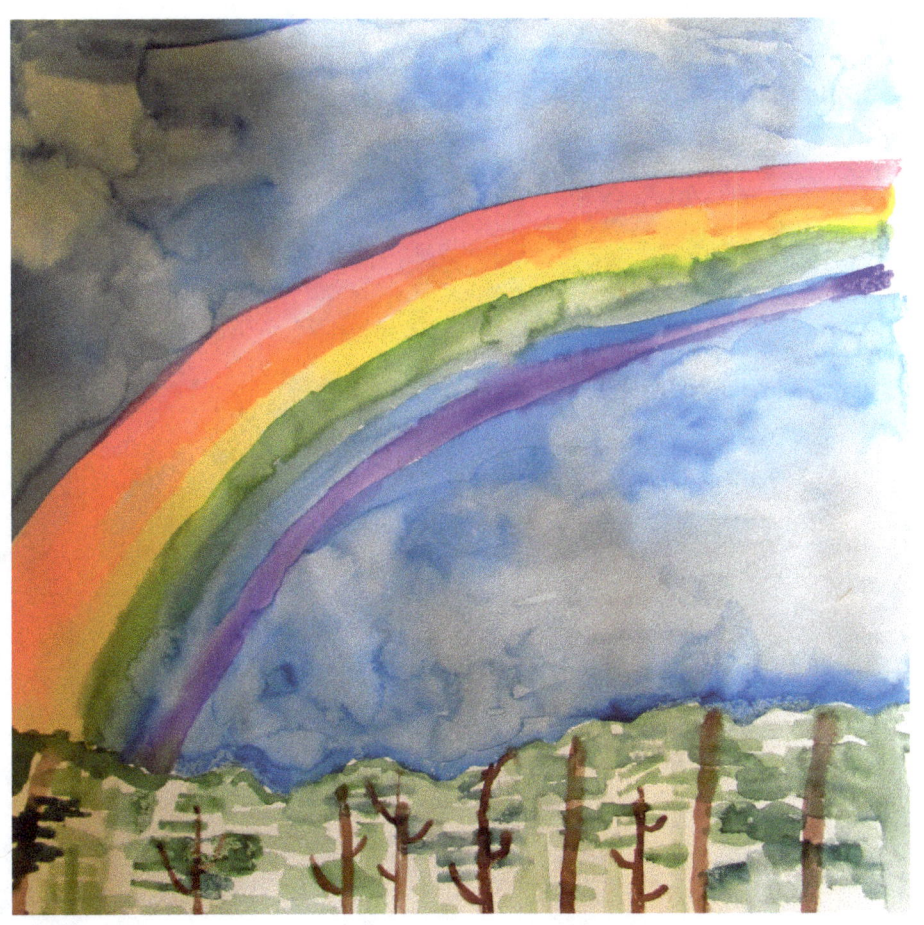

Prelude

The main thing is to be moved, to love, to hope, to tremble, to live.
—AUGUSTE RODIN

It's not what you look at that matters, it's what you see.
—HENRY DAVID THOREAU

SUNDAY, SEPTEMBER 22, 2007. The memorial service for my father had ended; the rest of the family and I had made our way to Chitwood Hall at First United Methodist Church of Tuscaloosa to receive many friends who had come to honor the life and legacy of Lester Eugene Potts, Jr. (November 4, 1928—September 15, 2007).

We gathered, surrounded by his beautiful art[1]—art created in the throes of Alzheimer's disease by someone who had never shown any such ability prior to the diagnosis. Art discovered at Caring Days,[2] a groundbreaking adult dementia daycare center where Lester had been hailed simply for being the Lester who walked through the door every day, a quantity of selfhood that was more than enough to make up for dementia-associated losses. Art that had been drawn forth from heart and mind by the able hands of

---

1. To view the watercolor art of Lester E. Potts, Jr., visit www.lesterslegacy.com.
2. Caring Days, part of the Mal and Charlotte Moore Center in Tuscaloosa, Alabama, is a day program for adults with Alzheimer's and other memory disorders. To learn more about their award-winning program, visit www.caringdays.org.

Part I: Prelude and Program Description

George Parker, a retired artist who had found his late-life calling bringing art to life from the fading memories of people living with dementia.

(I don't recall who actually told me the next part of the story; it may have been George himself. Perhaps the luster of it blurs my memory. Nevertheless, I relate it to you as truth.)

George had fallen on tough times, lying comatose in an intensive care unit somewhere between earth's shipwrecked shores and heaven's harbor docks. The crusty old artist, salted with sea spray from pondering how sunbeams strike the bricks of lighthouses so that he could shade his own works most expressively, had heard a voice within a great and glowing brightness telling him it was not his time, that he was being saved to share his artistic gift with people who were losing themselves in the sloughs of forgetfulness.

He awoke from this ineffable state with purpose undocked, some sand from the other shore in his hands, and his face shining like a Cecil B. "Demille-ified" Heston descending from Mount Sinai clutching tablets etched with a holy decree.

It so happened that Caring Days sought to start an art program for its clients near the time George had recovered enough to move about. Through an outreach initiative at a local community college, George was paired with Caring Days, and the rest is history, preserved in vibrant creations of client artists with whom he worked for several years. One of those folks was a sawmiller named Lester from rural Pickens County, Alabama, a utilitarian child of the Great Depression[3] who was known to move through art museums with the stealth and speed of a spy plane while his wife and son pondered every caption and brushstroke displayed therein.

It had been a treacherous crossing toward safe harbor at Caring Days. Dad was an otherwise healthy and very strong man of seventy when he started showing early signs. Misplaced memories. Fender benders. Vanishing keys. Turbulence in those still, deep pools of the self. Headwaters broke when he lost his job parking cars at a local office building because he couldn't find them—that is, cars, keys, coworkers, and himself. He, the near-perfect employee, the one who could outwork strapping youths, the dependable one who always did his work and saw to it that others got theirs done, too, no longer could hold his own.

Worst of all was the day he called to say his employment had ended. Somehow, this had a greater negative impact on me than the day he was

---

3. To view a short documentary from UAB about Lester's story and art, see UAB Magazine, "Painting in Twilight."

Prelude

diagnosed, the day we had to place him in a nursing home, the day of his commitment through probate court for being a danger to himself and others, even the day he passed away . . . Sometimes, the first among successive deaths is the most painful. And this was not about me. It hurt so badly because I imagined how much it must have pained him to admit that he no longer was employable. That he no longer was able to provide. That he couldn't safeguard his family against the ruin that, for children of the Depression, always lurked just past that last paycheck. And to see him losing the part of his identity that was anchored to his occupation.

Things got rough for a time after that. His progression was rapid. The kindest, gentlest man I've ever known was becoming hard to handle due to the disease. It was taking a toll on Mother, though she was doing a laudable job, as she loved him deeply through all of his pain, and hers.

Help came in the form of a faith-based dementia daycare center, Caring Days, Vicki Kerr, its executive director, and a wonderful group of board members, staff, and volunteers. Telling Dad that Caring Days needed workers to help make some repairs, we had no trouble getting him to agree to go down and help. From his moment of entry, hammer in hand, Dad was loved and accepted for being who he was in the present, not held to an unfair standard of who others expected him to be. After all, he was the same person he always had been, created, loved, and named by the God who had come to be his dearest friend, who was choosing with every breath to sustain his beautiful life to share with others and who would faithfully love and care for him, though the possibility loomed that the canvas of his mind might one day be erased.

Dad became very close to Vicki, who figured out how to survive his rib-crushing hugs by getting him to throw and catch kisses instead, and who, at the end of her eulogy at Dad's memorial service, symbolically reached up and caught one last kiss thrown from the front porch of his heavenly mansion. I remember saying to Vicki soon after Dad started attending Caring Days that I wished she had known him when he was "still my Dad." She shook her head and replied, "No, that's not the way it works here. We are going to love the Lester we greet when he gets here every day. That's the real Lester." I think that was the beginning of my enlightenment regarding the persistence of personhood despite dementia and the compassionate care we are compelled to give based on the truth of that realization. I am grateful beyond measure for that.

Part I: Prelude and Program Description

Before long, Dad would meet George Parker, whom I consider to be the "Anne Sullivan" to Dad's "Helen Keller." Though I was not there for the breakthrough moment when the gift finally showed itself (when blind, deaf, and mute, Helen finally understood what was meant by the word "w-a-t-e-r"[4]), I certainly saw the results. "W-a-t-e-r" colors of unbelievable depth and expressivity came pouring out, many of which seemed to tap into deeply submerged memories of childhood. Saws, high-topped shoes, logs on end, birdhouses, smokehouses, even his father's hat appeared on canvases as vibrantly colored as one would imagine Lewis Carroll's Wonderland to be. The beauty of the art and its impact on the viewer defy description. No one could believe it, especially those who had known Dad for many years. When our young daughters would say, "My Papa is an artist," those who had grown up with him often would reply, befuddled, "We must be talking about a different Lester Potts."

The art rescued him, in many ways, like a beacon from one of George's lighthouses. Because of the language loss associated with Alzheimer's disease, Lester no longer could tell his story in conventional ways. We all have an enduring need to share our stories. So, George helped him to paint it, and I believe that comforted Dad greatly. The part I could not see, however—the relationships that developed between George and the client artists and between the clients themselves as they were making art together—may have been the main transformative force, as we will describe later.

Dad's newfound creativity not only helped him, but its effects spilled over into the lives of others. He became less of a challenge to care for at home, his mood—and, therefore, the moods of those around him—improved, and the art had a powerfully inspirational effect on any who would stop to take a look. Dad loved showing it off and would eagerly lead guests into the living room repetitively to admire some of his favorites. The pride instilled into a broken life set him beaming. In fact, this is what Vicki says gave her and her Caring Days colleagues the most joy: "Giving a strong man something for which to be proud."

To be fair, I'll note that the art was made possible, in part, by the supportive, familiar, affirming, and safe environment of Caring Days. In order for that kind of vulnerability to be expressed and for those relationships to develop, Dad must have felt very comfortable and supported there.

---

4. Penn, *Miracle Worker*. For more depth on the story of Alabama's Helen Keller and Anne Sullivan, see the 1962 film *The Miracle Worker* at https://www.imdb.com/title/tt0056241/.

Prelude

Another way to say it might be that through excellent care, they actually *incubated his personhood* and enabled it to be born again through art and relationships. How do you adequately thank someone for doing that for your loved one?

I had not handled Dad's illness well. A neurologist and only child, I felt like I was failing my parents because I couldn't mitigate Dad's disability and I didn't have the knowledge or the experience by which to help Mother in the day-to-day challenges of caregiving. Stress, lack of sleep, and poor choices took a toll on my body and mind, but mostly on my spirit. My family suffered through this dark time, much darker because of the maladaptive way in which I handled it. I must confess, I have guilt in admitting this. Dad and Mother were going through much worse. But this is the toxicity of Alzheimer's. It leads each one into his or her own particular hell, then leaves them there, lost and forgotten.

Ironically, Dad's art (and my wife) rescued me as well. On a whim, my wife, Ellen, gave me an anthology of poetry written by Henry van Dyke,[5] and reading his words moved me deeply. I began to write. Before long, I was composing a poem a day, though I knew very little about writing poetry. After about a month of staying up every night writing poems, and with Ellen wondering what kind of beast she had unleashed, I asked if she thought we should publish a book of Dad's art and my poetry. She said, "Of course we should. Let's call it *The Broken Jar*." We decided to self-publish it[6] and offer the book to Caring Days in gratitude for all the wonderful things they had done for Dad and our family.

Through that book, some Caring Days art shows, and other publications and news media that had picked up the story of Dad's art, he became a regional celebrity of sorts. I am sure this must have been pleasing to George, though I never spoke with him about it. But this whole thing was gaining energy . . . it was such a reservoir of hope for many lives that were drying up in the deserts of dementia. Often, I have wondered if George sensed this happening—the energy of new life springing out of Lester's art—and thought back on his own resurrection and the calling he had received from deep within the luminous darkness of that experience.

Now, let's get back to that Sunday afternoon in September of 2007. From my place in the visitation line, I could see George. A diminutive

---

5. Van Dyke, *Poems*.

6. A few copies of *The Broken Jar* remain and are available at Caring Days in Tuscaloosa, Alabama (www.caringdays.org).

Part I: Prelude and Program Description

man, rough on the edges and long in the tooth, he hunkered back behind a couple of larger folks. He was dressed in a sport coat and tie in which he looked a bit shroud-bound but through which his light beams on the bay shone all over that room. The closer he got, the clearer I could see a sparkle in his eyes and the faint smile of one who knew part of a secret and couldn't wait to share the excitement with others.

The time came to thank George for what he had done for Dad, and I did so, profusely and with as much heart and humility as I could muster. I will never forget his response. With a wink and the aforementioned glint, he leaned in and whispered, "Son, you haven't seen anything yet. You just wait." And with that, he offered condolences and was on his way.

I never got an opportunity to ask George what he meant or even to see him again. He died a few short weeks later, his earthly mission accomplished. But I think I now know, at least in part, what he was alluding to.

The art and the story continued to gain notoriety after Dad's death. And my desire to find some way to pay it forward grew in equal measure. The American Academy of Neurology, mostly because of Dad's story and *The Broken Jar*, asked me to train to be an advocate for patients, caregivers, and my profession in the award-winning Donald Palatucci Advocacy Leadership Training program (PALF),[7] through which I gained valuable skills for more effective advocacy. As part of this program, each advocate must develop an action plan, something upon which to focus advocacy efforts and which could begin to have a measurable impact within one year. My action plan was to give the expressive arts more widespread use among persons living with dementia and their care partners, having witnessed the benefits this offered to Dad. Thus, the seed of what would grow into the Bringing Art to Life program was beginning to germinate.

In the PALF program, I was fortunate to meet impassioned, accomplished advocates like Dr. Elizabeth Barber, who later would arrange a digital art gallery showing of the art of her mother and my father at Chicago's National Museum of Health and Medicine. This event springboarded collaborations with a virtual reality company (Embodied Labs),[8] an eldercare company (Chicago Methodist Senior Services), and my friend and colleague Dr. Neelum Aggarwal, a Rush University cognitive neurologist,

---

7. For more on the American Academy of Neurology's Donald M. Palatucci Advocacy Leadership Training Program, see "Palatucci Advocacy Leadership."

8. Embodied Labs virtual reality training forms a core educational element for students in Bringing Art to Life. To learn more about Embodied Labs, visit https://embodiedlabs.com/.

who would be the lead faculty and visionary developer for Bringing Art to Life-Chicago, facilitated by two of our former BATL-Tuscaloosa students, Angela Ray and Cyrus Alavi.

Inspired by PALF and the passion and stories of other advocates, I came back home and worked hard to bring the action plan to fruition. First, a nonprofit foundation, Cognitive Dynamics,[9] was created, with a mission to improve quality of life for those living with dementia and their care partners through the expressive arts and storytelling. Soon afterward, another PALF advocate and friend, Los Angeles neurologist Dr. Meril Platzer, put us in contact with David W. Streets, a well-known art-gallery owner and art appraiser in Beverly Hills. He expressed keen interest in Dad's art and offered the opportunity to have an art gala at his gallery[10] to raise Alzheimer's/dementia awareness. The event took place on November 5, 2010, and was the flagship event for our foundation.

Shortly after this, my wife, Ellen, and I cowrote *A Pocket Guide for the Alzheimer's Care Giver*,[11] drawing from our experience with Dad and several other family members and other resources we had found helpful. David Streets connected us to Maria Shriver's organization, and Ms. Shriver endorsed our book and offered us the opportunity to blog about caregiving on her website as two of her Architects of Change.[12]

About this same time, a well-known art therapist, Angel Duncan,[13] having heard about Dad's story, reached out with a phone call and eventually traveled to Alabama. Out of this meeting and burgeoning friendship came plans to create an expressive arts program for persons living with dementia that also would provide educational opportunities for students. Further meetings with friends at the University of Alabama Honors College, primarily Dr. Jacqueline Morgan and Dr. Shane Sharpe, resulted in an opportunity to offer a class through which students of diverse majors would be paired with persons living with dementia, experiencing weekly art therapy sessions, developing relationships, and preserving life story details of their dementia partners. One of the university's most outstanding

---

9. To learn more about the nonprofit Cognitive Dynamics, visit www.cognitivedynamics.org.

10. To learn more about the David W. Streets Gallery showing of Lester Potts's art, see CognitiveDynamics1, "Bringing Art to Life."

11. Potts, *Pocket Guide*.

12. See "Caregiving."

13. Visit the website of Angel C. Duncan, executive arts director of Cognitive Dynamics Foundation (https://duncanangel.wixsite.com/angelcduncan).

Part I: Prelude and Program Description

students, Meg McCrummen (Fowler), was selected to be a student facilitator and further developer of the program, and Bringing Art to Life (UH 300 Art to Life), seeded by the life and art of Lester Potts, was brought to a bloom in the spring semester of 2011.

Having completed our tenth year, BATL has continued its presence in Tuscaloosa and has expanded to Chicago, Illinois, and Birmingham, Alabama, involving both high school and college students paired with persons living with dementia either in adult day programs or assisted living specialty-care units and facilitated by medical students. Original research has documented some of the program's benefits, a manual of implementation has been written, and plans are underway to expand the program into other areas.

Innovations from BATL-Chicago include the expanded use of virtual-reality training for medical students and certified nursing assistants (CNAs) who work with persons living with dementia, a sensory garden for participants and students, and a "Chai and Chat" educational discussion for parents of high school students involved in the program, part of an outreach to the Southeast Asian community. Additionally, spin-offs of the program include Crimson Community Café, Tuscaloosa's first memory café, and Art to Life Outreach, a service-learning opportunity for individual students to visit and do art projects with residents living with dementia in residential care settings or their homes, currently in Tuscaloosa and New Orleans, Louisiana. For the last several years at the Tuscaloosa location, the art therapy part of the program has taken place at Caring Days with their clients. This is very special to me, for obvious reasons, providing a means of saying, "Thank you for loving my father."

The students that have come through BATL are deeply impacted through relationships with their dementia partners, and we have been told that the program is one of the most transformative classes offered at the University of Alabama. Often, I tell people that all I would need to do for the program to be effective is to hold the door open for students to walk in and meet their dementia partners, because that is where the magic happens. Where lives are changed.

We are indebted to the art therapists—first, Angel Duncan, as well as Sarah Margaret Wade, Karen Gibbons, Amy Brown, Carrie Ezell, Millie Dawson-Hardy, Ally DeSantis, and Meredith Schroeder—who have guided us so effectively during our art therapy sessions. And I could not have run the program without the skill, dependability, hearts, and minds of some of

Prelude

the brightest lights in my circle of relationships: student facilitators Meg McCrummen Fowler, Emily Broman Phelps, Jacquelynn Myrick Dunn, Maggie Holmes, and Zoe Berndt in Tuscaloosa, and Angela Ray and Cyrus Alavi, who had the vision, passion, and dedication to start our program in Chicago (BATL-Chicago), as well as Art to Life Outreach facilitators Abby Holland, Madi Woo, and Morgan Roberts.

The quote at the beginning of this section of the book, which is commonly attributed to Thoreau, says, "It's not what you look at that matters, it's what you see."[14] When I looked at Dad after he developed Alzheimer's, I often saw a confused, disoriented, agitated, ashamed, and frightened man. But Caring Days, George Parker, and the art changed that. Sure, there were days even after Dad started painting in which the above characteristics were displayed, but much less often.

In general, the art and the care received at Caring Days helped Dad to live well in spite of the illness, to make meaning of even the parts of his life affected by disease. And we were enabled to see something different; gazing past the staring façade, we could see the colors of his soul—the enduring, beautiful, expressive person of Lester Potts fluttering out like the rainbow-colored hummingbird that was his first painting. Seeing him this way completely changed my medical practice. Because of the experience with Dad, I now try to do a better job of honoring personhood and innate dignity no matter how advanced the disease. I seek out relationships with those who are living with dementia and their caregivers and try never to write off someone because of their disability, regardless of what it may be.

All of this has made me a better person—a better physician, a better teacher, and a better care partner—and, to quote a mentor, Dr. James M. Houston, "has brought things out of me that are potentials for my own growth."[15] I hope and pray that through this book, I am able to share some of the things I have learned for the upbuilding of others.

Now for a word about this book. It is not a how-to manual for Bringing Art to Life, and it is not a scientific/academic publication through which to elaborate on research findings, though those will be mentioned. The book is the venue through which I hope to share lessons learned over the past ten

14. Thoreau, "It's Not What . . ."

15. Personal communication. The life, writings, philosophy, faith, and friendship of Dr. James M. Houston have had a major impact on Bringing Art to Life. To learn more about his thoughts on personhood and care partnership with his late wife, Rita, see CognitiveDynamics1, "Personhood in Dementia," for an interview conducted at his home in Vancouver in 2012 (part of the educational curriculum of Bringing Art to Life).

Part I: Prelude and Program Description

years from persons living with cognitive disorders, their care partners, art therapists with whom I have worked, guest faculty, volunteers and sources, and the marvelous students who have come through our program—essential lessons about what it means to be a human being, alive to whatever conditions in which we find ourselves. In the following pages, stories will be shared of individuals who have participated in the program (names will be changed to protect the identities of the persons involved), along with descriptions of various elements of our philosophy of care and how they emerged from experiences we have had in this program.

Additionally, I hope to share another gift the program has offered. In the beacon lights from the faces of clients living with dementia, caregivers, and students, I have come alive to myself—the true self, that person who exists in relationship to God, others, and the cosmos. Rodin is credited for saying, "The main thing is to be moved, to love, to hope, to tremble, to live."[16] And it is only through this enlivened and embodied personhood that I have any chance at all of helping others. So, part of the story will be my own tale of growth and revelation charting through the channels of this narrative.

Finally, and most importantly, I want to honor the love, compassion, providence, and calling of God, first made manifest in near-death experiences—George's, Dad's, even mine—and continuing to be expressed through every chapter of this story. As long as we can remain in the stream of that energetic flow, I feel that the program will continue to be effective in its mission to provide quality and meaning to lives, and the story will live itself out in others, bringing art to life for years to come.

---

16. Rodin, "The Main Thing . . ."

BATL Program Description

Creativity nurtures the brain.
—ANGEL C. DUNCAN,
executive arts director, Cognitive Dynamics Foundation

BRINGING ART TO LIFE (BATL)[1] is a service-learning program developed by the Cognitive Dynamics Foundation in memory of Lester E. Potts, Jr. Its primary purpose is to honor and validate persons living with dementia and other cognitive disorders through art therapy, other expressive arts, and storytelling. Additional goals include facilitating the development of intergenerational, multicultural relationships; growing empathy, compassion, knowledge, and self-awareness in students via transformational educational paradigms; lessening stigma; providing respite for care partners; and laying a foundation for the ongoing engagement and enrichment of students, persons living with dementia, and their care partners in the broader community.

The program accepts anywhere from ten to twenty college undergraduate or high school students per semester. Many, but not all, of these students have a family member who is living with dementia, and most are pursuing careers in health care. After a few weeks of education and training, the students are paired, usually two or three to one, with persons living with dementia who either are residents in specialty-care assisted-living facilities or who are participants in adult day programs.

1. The website for Bringing Art to Life may be viewed here: https://www.cognitivedynamics.org/bringing-art-to-life/.

Part I: Prelude and Program Description

The educational program includes comprehensive lectures from neurologists about the neuroscience of memory, Alzheimer's disease, and other dementias, including subjects such as epidemiology, pathophysiology, common clinical manifestations and their pathophysiological correlations, diagnosis and imaging, methods of cognitive assessment, prevention, treatment, and updates on research. Additionally, students are trained on methods of interacting with persons who have dementia and participate in simulated, first-person, embodied dementia experiences via the Virtual Dementia Tour from Second Wind Dreams and virtual-reality training modules from Embodied Labs. Lectures on the history, theory, and practice of art therapy and a discussion of art therapy directives to be used is offered, as well as lectures on caregiving.

Mindfulness training is provided primarily as a means of enhancing the relational impact of the art therapy sessions through better listening, enhanced capacity for compassion and empathy, increased self-awareness, and as a check against prejudgments and emotional reactivity. Also, it may provide students with a new lens to engage experiences which may prove beneficial to their wellness later in their lives and careers.

An extensive list of required and optional readings is included to support learning. Examples include research publications about the effectiveness of art therapy interventions in dementia populations; guidelines offered to physicians on helping dementia patients to live well; ethical perspectives on stigma, personhood, and the toxicity of the tragedy narrative of dementia (the negative lens through which dementia typically is considered) on perceived quality of life; methods of life review; first-person dementia narratives; etc.

Media presentations, including documentaries such as *I Remember Better When I Paint* (Hilgos Foundation),[2] *Do You Know Me Now?* (Cognitive Dynamics Foundation),[3] and *Alive Inside* (Alive Inside Foundation),[4] help students understand the power of the expressive arts to tap into personhood, build relationships, combat stigma, enhance quality of life, and build supportive communities for persons living with dementia. Care-partner training videos also are shared, as well as other online media

---

2. Ellena and Huebner, *I Remember Better*. To learn more about *I Remember Better When I Paint*, visit http://www.hilgos.org/.

3. See CognitiveDynamics1, "Do You Know Me Now?"

4. Rossato-Bennett, *Alive Inside*. To learn more about *Alive Inside*, visit http://www.aliveinside.us/#land.

BATL Program Description

addressing the science of Alzheimer's and the other dementias, empathy and compassion, the expressive arts, and mindfulness. Taped interviews from such sources as Cathie Borrie (author of *The Long Hello*[5]); Naomi Feil (person-centered care pioneer and founder of The Validation Method[6]); friends and fellow advocates Lynda Everman (Alzheimer's semipostal-stamp champion and creator of the Alzheimer's Stole Ministry and Tallit Initiative[7]) and Don Wendorf (psychologist, musician, and author[8]); the Reverend Dr. Richard Morgan (a pastor and author whose book *Treasure for Alzheimer's* shares the art of Lester Potts and stories of how Dr. Morgan used the art to communicate with persons in late-stage dementia[9]); and philosopher and theologian Dr. James M. Houston deepen understanding and promote discussion. Students are encouraged to read and write poetry, create and view art, listen to music, tap into imagination, and explore dance and movement as avenues to a better understanding of the human response to cognitive decline and other disorders, as a means to build resiliency, to hone listening and observation skills, and to further refine personal acumen of empathy and compassion.

Several student creative writing assignments are given during the semester, encompassing topics such as writing a memoir about a significant interaction with an elderly person or someone living with dementia, an essay about what they plan to give of themselves to the BATL experience, a poem about a piece of artwork created by their dementia partner, and an essay based on the assumption that they themselves have dementia, are moving into a nursing home, and must write a letter to their care partners telling them what they should know to enable the provision of person-centered care. Furthermore, students write weekly journals about the art therapy experience of the preceding week, their thoughts regarding a particular source they have read, or their impressions of the embodied dementia training.

---

5. Borrie, *Long Hello*.

6. The philosophy, teachings, and approach of dementia-care pioneer Naomi Feil have greatly influenced the educational curriculum and caregiving paradigm of Bringing Art to Life. To learn more about Naomi Feil and her pioneering work through The Validation Institute, visit https://vfvalidation.org/.

7. To learn more about Lynda Everman's Alzheimer's Stole Ministry and Tallit Initiative, read Everman and Wendorf, *Stolen Memories*.

8. Wendorf, *Caregiver Carols*.

9. Morgan and Potts, *Treasure for Alzheimer's*.

Part I: Prelude and Program Description

Ongoing research at the BATL-Tuscaloosa location conducted by a team from the Alabama Research Institute on Aging (ARIA) under the leadership of University of Alabama geropsychologist Dr. Rebecca Allen[10] has shown that students in BATL experience increases in empathy and improved attitudes toward older adults and persons living with dementia. Additionally, compared to students in psychology of aging or introductory psychology courses, BATL students demonstrated improved attitudes toward individuals living with dementia.[11] Existential awareness appears to foster mindfulness and empathy that subsequently facilitate these changes in ageist attitudes.[12] Engagement with group members in the present moment has been found to be a more powerful predictor of intergenerational relationship building than meaningful engagement with art.[13] Two emergent themes identified in present moment verbal engagements were validation of personhood and reminiscence of family ties.[14] These results suggest that experiential learning opportunities like BATL are critical to infusing enthusiasm for intergenerational collaborations, possibly influencing students' future career trajectories and motivating desire to work with older adults.

Our BATL-Chicago team, under the leadership of Dr. Neelum Aggarwal, has assessed the effects of a modified version of the program tailored to a group of multicultural, multiracial Certified Nursing Assistant (CNA) staff at a specialty-care assisted-living facility and found that BATL participants reported greater levels of insight and empathy while working with their residents, citing the immersive virtual reality curriculum as influential.[15] Participants expressed an appreciation for the opportunity to have access to both a cognitive neurologist and a neuropsychologist to ask questions about specific patients and receive advice on techniques for dealing with challenging dementia-related behavior.[16] This project shows promise in leveraging virtual reality and other empathy-enhancing training to teach

---

10. To learn more about Rebecca S. Allen, professor of psychology and director of the Alabama Research Institute on Aging, see "Rebecca S. Allen."
11. Allen and Carden, "Bridging the Past."
12. Reel et al., "Bringing Art to Life," 1.
13. Reel et al., "Bringing Art to Life," 1.
14. Reel et al., "Bringing Art to Life," 1.
15. Balas and Aggarwal, "Training Curriculum."
16. Shaw et al., "Enhancing Dementia Care."

BATL Program Description

CNAs dementia curriculum from a patient-perspective orientation, in addition to improving their foundational dementia knowledge.[17]

BATL-associated research has been presented at numerous national and international meetings, including Alzheimer's Association International Conferences,[18] Gerontological Society of America symposia,[19] and the World Congress of the International Association for Gerontology and Geriatrics,[20] and two papers have been published as of the printing of this book, with more to come.[21] BATL faculty are active internationally in dementia advocacy circles, are frequent guests on blogs and podcasts, are keynote speakers in conferences, and author numerous articles incorporating the themes and care philosophies of BATL. In future iterations of the program, we plan to increase our focus on the assessment of art therapy's and virtual reality's impact on outcomes.

---

17. Shaw et al., "Enhancing Dementia Care."
18. Ivey et al., "Intergenerational Service-Learning Experience."
19. Allen and Carden, "Bridging the Past."
20. Ivey et al., "Intergenerational Service-Learning Experience."
21. Reel et al., "Bringing Art to Life"; Balas and Aggarwal, "Training Curriculum."

Building a Culture of Compassion

> Because you are not what I would have you be,
> I blind myself to who, in truth, you are.
> —MADELEINE L'ENGLE

> All paths lead to the same goal: to convey to others what we are.
> —PABLO NERUDA

PROOF THAT AN EXPERIENCE was vital, real, and true lies in its lasting impact on us and others around us, including its power to consistently produce a sense of gratitude and drive future behavior for the good. Such has been the experience reported by those of us involved in BATL.

Over the past ten years, it has been my privilege to closely observe the relationships that have developed between some 300 college and high school students of diverse majors and approximately 150 persons living with dementia with whom they have been paired in our program. I believe the transformative nature of the BATL experience is due, primarily, to these relationships.

Students in BATL are encouraged to espouse the belief/creed that *each person has innate value and dignity despite conditions or circumstances; that personhood is inherent and unfading, despite any inability of ours to perceive it.* This creed colors everything we do in BATL, and we believe it is the framework upon which all models of care should be built.

Enlightened with a better understanding of the pathophysiology and clinical manifestations of the condition and given the tools to aid in listening and communicating—along with practice in creating safe and open encounters characterized by vulnerability, present moment-centeredness, and non-judgment through the practice of mindfulness and presence—students are ready to meet their dementia partners. During the ensuing sessions, students work to build a supportive environment for participants. This enables the expression of personhood through creativity, engagement of imagination, connection with true selfhood, and sharing of stories.

As described in the preceding chapter, the students' educational experience is designed to set the stage for deep encounters with persons living with dementia of the type philosopher Martin Buber described as "I-Thou," rather than "I-It" encounters.[1] Buber considered this type of encounter as a revelation of presence, a transcendent concept of mutuality occupying the space between separate entities, in which they are found to be in relationship.[2] There can be no objectification or diminishment of the other in such a relationship, because the essence of the other, just as the essence of oneself, is seen as inviolate. "In every You, we address the eternal You," says Buber.[3] I believe this alludes to the particle of pure indwelling identity deep within each human being, which, when beheld, is apt to move one to a state of gratitude, awe, and wonder. Relational energies flow naturally in these conditions.

We all have a life story to share. Poet Maya Angelou has said that "there is no greater agony than bearing an untold story inside you."[4] Dementia, through its effects on verbal expression and its impact on maintaining a congruent past, present, and future narrative, can adversely impact an individual's ability to share her story. The process of art therapy in the relational milieu described above promotes story sharing, reminiscence, and life review, and the students are instructed to take note of all the life story elements that are revealed during the sessions. Gathering information and forming a gestalt through which to know an individual more intimately are essential elements of compassionate person-centered care.

Rather than trying to acquire only factual data (which can be challenging and even frustrating), the students are encouraged to try to understand

1. Buber, *I and Thou*, 75–76.
2. Buber, *I and Thou*, 75–76.
3. Buber, *I and Thou*, 56.
4. Angelou, *Caged Bird Sings*, 74.

Part I: Prelude and Program Description

who the person is with whom they are interacting each week: What are his likes and dislikes? Who and what does she love, and who loves her? What is her personality type? What would he do on his favorite day? How has getting to know and appreciate this person impacted you as a student? These and other elements form the building blocks of the LifeBio.com[5] legacy books or life scrapbooks the students produce for their participants at the end of the semester and lay the framework for the relationships that continue long after the sessions come to a close.

All of us have character traits that, for the most part, persist throughout our lives. Persons living with dementia continue to have these as well, though they may be harder to identify through the progression of cognitive impairment. In BATL, we call these persistent self traits "pillars of personhood,"[6] and we seek to find them in each of our participants, building relationships upon them during our time together. This search for the elements of personhood fosters the provision of compassionate, dignifying, affirming care for those living with dementia and nurtures the kind of relationships we are seeking. In addition, it helps to mitigate pervasive stigma against those living with dementia, which I believe is based upon negation of personhood and resultant abandonment of opportunities for relationship building and "I-Thou" encounters previously described.

Near the end of the art therapy sessions, we meet together for an in-depth discussion about the personhood of each of our participants, and we identify and discuss their pillars in four categories: physical, psychological, spiritual, and relational. After these discussions, we feel we have as good a handle as possible on the breadth and depth of who these people are and are in a better position to accomplish the noble and challenging work of showing them back to themselves through their own stories, into which we have been woven.

This process is facilitated by the gift of person-centered quilts by our friend and fellow advocate Lynda Everman, in collaboration with the Alzheimer's Study Quilt Project.[7] This project, an initiative of the Alzheimer's Disease Cooperative Study (ADCS), sponsored by the University of California, San Diego, accepts quilt donations from quilters across the country, which are then given to study participants in gratitude for their

5. See https://secure.lifebio.com/.

6. For a discussion of pillars of personhood, see Vaillancourt, "Pillars of Personhood."

7. To read more about the the Alzheimer's Study Quilt Project and the Alzheimer's Disease Cooperative Study, see "Alzheimer's Study Quilt Project."

involvement. Lynda Everman collects pillars-of-personhood information from the students, which she then uses to create unique life-story quilts for each of our BATL participants or passes on to the ADCS for them to select appropriate quilts. Fabric holds memories, and these quilts preserve and honor their life histories. We see this as another way to help our participants raise a banner of their own colors again, even as dementia tries to fly the flag of their valedictory surrender.

The directives (activities, projects) planned by the art therapists are designed to facilitate expression and are coupled with reminiscence, with attention to emotional memories and meaningful past relationships the participants have had. At times, the participants may have some difficulty or lack of interest with the directives, or they may prefer to share stories or observe others during the art therapy sessions. Flexibility to allow such spontaneous expression is encouraged. Likewise, the imaginations of the participants and students are allowed free expression within the safe space of the art therapy environment. And the engagement with art, especially in such a supportive space, taps into the autobiographical memories of our partners who are living with dementia, as has been described in the art therapy literature.[8]

Sessions often start with simple mindfulness activities, with the goal of centering everyone in the present moment. As mentioned, students are encouraged to practice non-judgment regarding the abilities or limitations of their participants and to focus on what the participants still can do. The process, not the outcome, is important. The end results of any creative activity are validated, but there is no expected product, and participants are not pressured to produce art.

Students learn to practice mindful listening, looking for nonverbal expression, and times of silent observation are encouraged. During these times of silence, as an observer I have sensed some of the most powerful communication occurring between the students and their participants, as well as with the other students in each small group.

Over the course of the semester, group dynamics begin to change. Those living with dementia become more comfortable and appear to be more trusting of the environment, even though some of them do not seem to remember the students who are working with them from week to week. But the change in freedom of expression provides evidence that on some

---

8. Hass-Cohen and Findlay, *Art Therapy*, 12.

level, there exists recall that is built upon progressively over the course of the semester.

The students are encouraged to open themselves up to share their own stories with their participants as well. It has been my observation that the persons living with dementia facilitate this sharing themselves by asking questions of the students. In fact, many of the participants take on a mentoring or teaching role during the art therapy directives by asking students to work on the project while the participant observes and offers guidance and encouragement. Generativity, one of Erik Erikson's stages of psychosocial development, is commonly expressed by participants in these sessions.[9]

Some of the most palpable relational energies are present in small groups in which the person living with dementia is more advanced and is lacking many of the verbal skills retained in those with milder impairment. I have been impressed with the students' intentionality and perception—how they pick up on subtle elements of communication that are occurring through artistic expression, posture, eye contact, silence, etc. In fact, students in small groups like this often have a greater understanding of what makes up the personhood of their participants than students who have worked with a person at an earlier stage of impairment. It is as if something unnamable within their dementia partner is calling out to the students in the silent space left by lost language, and something unnamable inside the students is awakened to respond. These observations have taught me so much about the art of forming and maintaining relationships with people at the later stages of dementia.

The relationships I've observed between the students and their participants are characterized by such qualities as spontaneity, imagination, non-judgment, silence, flow, safety, humor, reciprocity, deference, validation, humility, kindness, encouragement, unconditionality, growth, and expansion.

As the persons living with dementia become more trusting and expressive in successive weeks, the student small groups undergo a change within themselves. The students often speak of how they are more willing to discuss their own struggles and imperfections with other members of their small group, and how they feel more comfortable being vulnerable and authentic—being "real"—after a few weeks. They speak of greater facility in mindfulness and an improved ability to center themselves in the present moment. There is a developing appreciation of the "little things" and a

---

9. For information about Erikson's stages of psychosocial development, see McLeod, "Stages of Psychosocial Development."

Building a Culture of Compassion

greater feeling of gratitude for life as it is. Students often speak of an honest appraisal of prejudices they have had about people who are old or have disabilities, even expressions of remorse and a desire to change. As mentioned in the last chapter, our BATL research team has shown that students show improvements in measures of empathy and ageist attitudes, as well as those measures reflecting stigma toward persons with dementia.

Students and participants alike show deference to each other; group dynamics assume a nurturing characteristic that flows naturally from trust, authenticity, empathy, and honest acceptance of imperfections. Mistakes are quickly forgiven, and humor and imagination find freedom of expression.

We make use of music in art therapy sessions as well. Led by fellow advocate Dr. Don Wendorf[10] and other friends, live music days are some of the most impactful sessions of each semester. Their participatory, mostly lively, and sometimes introspective nature creates an atmosphere of warm expressivity which carries over into subsequent weeks of art therapy, opening up BATL relationships at a greater depth. The response of the participants and their student groups has been amazing, as subsequent stories will show.

The music facilitates expression not only of joy but also, at times, of sadness or melancholy. On one occasion, Cara, a ninety-year-old living with moderate Alzheimer's, became somewhat moved during the music and spontaneously reached for the hand of one of her students. This was a giant leap for Cara, who, up to that time, had been somewhat reserved in the art therapy sessions. This had no small impact on the student and forged a deep intergenerational connection between the two of them that provided a foundation for the rest of the semester.

At the end-of-semester celebration, when the students present framed art, person-centered quilts, and either legacy books (from LifeBio.com) or scrapbooks to their participants and their families, the students stand up and tell their participants what the experience of working with them and getting to know them has meant. This is one of the most poignant parts of the program, as the students' heartfelt comments show just how deeply they have been impacted through the relationships. They also have learned so much about themselves, have learned to be more compassionate with themselves, and have developed deeper connections with their core humanity.

---

10. Dr. Don Wendorf has created sing-along music videos that are particularly appropriate for persons living with dementia and care partners, accessible on YouTube. He has also written a blog on how to do sing-alongs that incorporates the basic principles of person-centered care, available by emailing him at don_wendorf@yahoo.com.

Part I: Prelude and Program Description

As was stated earlier, often I tell people that all I would need to do to facilitate a transformative experience for the students in this program is to hold open the door leading to the art therapy room, because it is through the relationships themselves, in the setting of creativity, imagination, freedom of expression, and fully lived and shared moments, that the transformation occurs.

Probing to the depth of anything yields the ore of pure presence, the hidden relational force that calls everyone to dance in the empty spaces of life. If only we will stop, trust, listen, be intentional, and learn to love what is right in front of us.

Something real, something true is happening in these relationships. I believe it has to do with the depth of the relational space shared, the mutual vulnerability and trust exhibited in those spaces/moments, and the purity and authenticity of the presence that characterizes these occasions.

Participants in these relationships, including mindful observers, often are transformed to the degree that they are willing to surrender to the phenomenon of being fully alive and undefended in the mutuality of the present moment. It seems to me that such experiences are rare these days.

To observe this holy unfolding is quite humbling and inspiring, and has removed any personal doubts that meaningful relationships can be maintained with people who are living with dementia at any stage.

Father Richard Rohr has said, "How one does anything is how one does everything."[11] If students can learn to bring their most virtuous human qualities to the table while interacting and forming relationships with people who have dementia, then perhaps these qualities will be more freely expressed in the whole of their lives.

This, I believe, helps to build a culture of compassion for all, including those who are living with cognitive disorders.

---

11. I heard Richard Rohr say this at the 2015 CONSPIRE conference presented by the Center for Action and Contemplation on July 10–12, 2015.

The Room

Service to others is the rent you pay for your room here on earth.
—MUHAMMAD ALI

I MUST CONFESS, I had not paid much attention to the press and praise surrounding the rap musical phenomenon *Hamilton*, though my daughters could sing every word by rote. Then one day, my wife, Ellen, and I appeased our girls during a road trip and listened to the soundtrack. Several times during the recording, I felt I would need to take the nearest exit and simply stop on the shoulder and cry, or try and get my mind around the power of the story and absolute genius and inspiration required to create such a work of art.

Like so many times before, my mind and its prejudgements had attempted to block an opportunity I'd been given to experience something new, to see something in a different light, or to have an encounter with something potentially transformative that I had no idea I needed. Not long after that, we acquired tickets to the show when it was playing in Chicago and had a wonderful weekend family trip. Now I am a big fan.

One of my favorite songs from the musical is about a secret meeting in which an unprecedented political compromise settled the location of the new nation's capitol in exchange for political support for Alexander Hamilton's financial plan. With a well-known preexisting phrase as its title, "The Room Where It Happens" alludes to the importance of what took place

Part I: Prelude and Program Description

there and the privilege of having been present for those discussions that would change the course of America and the lives of its citizens.[1]

In BATL, "the room where it happens"—where the lives of the program's participants are transformed—is at Tuscaloosa's Caring Days Adult Daycare (the Mal and Charlotte Moore Center).

Through the years, Caring Days has allowed us to partner with them in BATL. Most of our participants in the Alabama iteration of the program have been clients at Caring Days, and we have held most of our weekly art therapy sessions there on Fridays. This is a privilege for which we are profoundly grateful, because we know what Caring Days is all about, and the atmosphere there sets the tone for the sessions.

In 1994, members of First Presbyterian Church of Tuscaloosa recognized the need for an adult daycare option for persons with cognitive disorders and began the work of forming a nonprofit, Caring Congregations, the parent entity for Caring Days, which now has grown to more than twenty congregations of different faiths. Opening its doors in 1997, Caring Days has been designated an "Excellence in Care, Dementia Program of Distinction" by the Alzheimer's Foundation of America, one of the few organizations in the United States to have received this honor.[2] A pass through the facility would convince anyone why they hold this accolade.

Caring Days is about people. Executive directors Vicki Kerr (founding) and LaDerrick Smith (current) are the heart and soul of the program and set the tone for the exemplary, dignifying care that occurs at Caring Days every minute of every day. They are surrounded by a staff of employees and volunteers that work wonders within this philosophy of care.

When my father attended Caring Days, they operated on part of one floor of the Easter Seals building in very close quarters. But, under the leadership of a capital campaign committee that had University of Alabama athletic director Mal Moore (former offensive coordinator for legendary football coach Paul "Bear" Bryant) as its honorary chair, Caring Days expanded into a beautiful new building of its own, greatly enlarging its community impact and enhancing the experience it could offer to clients and their families. Coach Moore had quietly and faithfully cared for his wife, Charlotte, during her twenty-year battle with Alzheimer's and had not known such a program existed. Thus, he and his family enthusiastically

---

1. Miranda and McCarter, *Hamilton the Revolution*, 158.

2. To learn more about the Excellence in Dementia Care Programs of Distinction, see "Excellence in Care."

The Room

supported the campaign for improved facilities and expanded services for Caring Days.

The building is one of the finest examples of dementia-friendly design I have seen; no detail has been neglected. And the facility is literally filled with art, from nature photography to client art to sculpture to the woodwork to the paintings of local professional artists, inspiring everyone by the beauty displayed.

Walking through the doors, one is comforted and held safely by the building and the art and friendly faces it contains. Everyone there seems happy and alive. No one sits alone in a corner. No one is left out. People are singing, playing, dancing, creating, laughing, and living. Who has dementia and who does not? One would be hard-pressed to tell.

Vicki put so much of herself into the building, choosing the art, supervising the design, etc. Most adult daycare centers are not able to take care of people when they reach the advanced stage of dementia, at which time most are transitioned into a nursing home or specialty-care assisted living facility. But Caring Days has committed to continue to serve their client population as far into the late stages as possible and has designed innovative and compassionate paradigms to keep those individuals engaged and living as well as they can.

At Caring Days, no one is forgotten, not even those who have passed away. Vicki commissioned an artist to create a mosaic of pieces of memorabilia from former clients. Whether they be bits of art, items of jewelry, or other keepsakes, these were incorporated into a beautiful and meaningful work of art that one passes on the way into the building. During each semester of BATL, when the students take their tour of Caring Days at the start of the semester, we make a stop by the mosaic at the end of the tour; I cherish anew the looks of wonder on their faces. And I always take the opportunity to show them a few little pieces of my father's ceramic trees that are embedded among the stations of hundreds of other lives memorialized there.

Not everyone knows that Vicki wrote the names of deceased clients on the framework of the building when it was under construction, so that everyone who had ever been a part of the program could be present in the new building, literally remembered within its very walls.

As I mentioned in the introduction to the book, I had not been present in the "room where it happened," where George Parker had worked with Dad and others those years ago. But, in attempting to create a similar experience through our program in the same facility that had meant so much to Dad and to our family, I hoped to be present to see a "brand new start" for others who "dream in the dark."[3] I wanted to be there and to bring others as well into the "room where it happens." A room with no stigma, no judgement, no requirement but love.

If it weren't for Caring Days and its founders, Vicki Kerr, LaDerrick Smith, and all the staff, clients, and families, there likely would have been no art of Lester Potts and no Bringing Art to Life program in his memory. And none of us would have been given the life-changing gift of being in the room where it happens.

We will never be able to adequately express our gratitude and appreciation for the people and place of Caring Days Adult Daycare Center.

---

3. Miranda and McCarter, *Hamilton the Revolution*, 190.

Thoughts on the Spiritual in Dementia Care

> We are not human beings having a spiritual experience.
> We are spiritual beings having a human experience.
> —PIERRE TEILHARD DE CHARDIN

THE CORE CREED OF Bringing Art to Life is that each person has innate value and dignity despite conditions or circumstances, and that personhood is inherent and unfading, despite any inability of ours to perceive it. Other than this, we officially espouse no particular religious position or dogma and make no requirements that students and participants in the program adopt a spiritual viewpoint or belief.

That said, in my quest to teach and mentor from a position of authenticity and the sharing of truth, I have no choice but to let my voyage through the seas of dementia, the stories of others whom I have been privileged to sail alongside, and the associated spiritual growth this has produced guide students in their own educational journeys. In the program, we hope our students will allow themselves to explore the depths of our shared humanity, and we leave it up to them to interpret their own experiences and to search for meaning therein.

The older I become, the more I see dementia care as a spiritual endeavor. Primarily, this is because most of the people whom I have observed to be living well either as persons diagnosed with dementia or care partners of those with dementia rely heavily on the spiritual for their sustenance and well-being and to make some kind of meaning of the experience. Also,

Part I: Prelude and Program Description

I credit others—clergy and faith leaders,[1] elders, mentors, professionals, mental health professionals and counselors, artists, writers, family members, etc.—who have helped to shape my own faith and spiritual beliefs and practices.

Here, I am employing a broad definition of the spiritual as having to do with the essential, the inner, the soulful, the relational, that which promotes growth and not decay, acceptance and not denial, peace as opposed to conflict, love as opposed to fear, trust as opposed to anxiety, gratitude in contrast to resentment, community as opposed to isolation, creativity as opposed to stagnation, depth instead of superficiality, compassion rather than heartlessness, other-centeredness rather than self-centeredness, and true-self orientation as opposed to ego-self orientation.

Honoring the spiritual in dementia care is about acknowledging the sacred core within each of us, that inviolate, imparted, incarnate entity which forms the central element of the self, rendering personhood immune to diminution by any state, condition, disease, decree, reductionistic definition, or philosophy.

Thus considered, personhood becomes the solid foundation upon which to build the structures of dementia care, with the goal of supporting this personhood, enabling its expression, and promoting its natural relational energies to build self- and others-supporting community. It can be found if we cultivate the perception to "see" it. I consider this to be spiritual work of high order.

Such a stance has a strong theological basis which is beyond the scope of this chapter. In his book *Dementia: Living in the Memories of God*, Dr. John Swinton speaks of persons living with dementia as being eternally remembered by God: "Despite confusion, true personal identity is known and held only by God, and nothing can destroy such divine recognition."[2] And, in their book *No Act of Love Is Ever Wasted*, authors Dr. Jane Thibault and the Reverend Dr. Richard Morgan posit that "at some level the person (with dementia) lives deeply in the mystery of God's love, in intimate connection with God's love, without the distractions of the world."[3] Thus, seeking the abiding self of one living with dementia is best considered in spiritual terms and within the spiritual framework of love.

---

1. Everman and Wendorf, *Dementia-Friendly Worship*, 9–12.
2. Swinton, *Dementia*, 218.
3. Morgan and Thibault, *Act of Love*, 30.

Thoughts on the Spiritual in Dementia Care

The benefits of considering the dementia journey and dementia care as spiritual may be self-evident, coalescing in the promotion of well-being: the reduction of stress and its effects, the fostering of resiliency, the making of meaning amidst suffering, the garnering of hope and joy despite loss and grief, the enabling of generativity despite growing dependence, and eventually, the cultivation of presence and transcendence—an unbinding, if you will, of dementia's restraints.

One may practice the spiritual in dementia care and not know it or, at least, not name it. There is nothing wrong with that. However, considering the spiritual as spiritual has some advantages. First, it brings an element of mystery, of ethereal goodness, which one may find to be supportive. This can promote trust in something greater than oneself and one's own powers, which may be taxed in care partnership. It can be exhausting to struggle, in futility, to exert one's power in attempts to control situations that cannot be controlled. Furthermore, considering the spiritual as spiritual may call forth a sense of awe or wonder, promoting humility and fostering gratitude. Additionally, it can create a sense of belonging or fitting into a much larger framework, a broader field, which can be a freeing and embracing experience.

The world of the spiritual is a world of gifts—graces small and large, often unexpected—which can bring uplifts on dark days and for which one may begin to look, expecting to find these hidden treasures in the secular and mundane. Sunbeams strike dewdrops suspended on a rose petal just past dawn. Some streetlight glows with warmth and brilliance upon a steel-gray sky. A mother holds her three children against the cold as they wait for the school bus, and you happen to see them on your way to work. Your mother, whom you suspect has forgotten you, calls you by your childhood nickname; again, you find the lost relationship in the light of her sparkling eyes. And you are grateful, and something inside you bows down.

Seeking the spiritual in dementia care means reaching for the depths of another person, coming into contact with the core of authenticity. In order to do this, one must find a way to access the same place in oneself, though I believe this initially is not the focus. I believe this inner journey is enabled through the care partnership, if allowed, and accompanied by openness, vulnerability, mindful listening, non-judgment, and reciprocity, so that one learns to receive energy and care from the relationship, consistent with the concept of growth versus decay that characterizes spirituality. This helps to guard against burnout. One learns to let the inner self of another minister to, energize, and inspire them. I believe one may even cultivate a sense of awe, as mentioned earlier, from encountering the depth of another person in this way, in spite of any losses that may be occurring on the exterior.

Layers with which society and culture have invested us seem to insulate us well from making contact of any depth with ourselves, our neighbors, or the intransient elements of our surroundings. Many of us seem to skim the surface of our existence, making few waves, and rarely encounter things that can truly change us and bring us to life. It seems great love or great suffering are required to awaken us.[4]

I believe persons who are living with dementia have shed some of those layers and often are living and interacting from a more authentic place than many of us who do not have dementia. In theory, this should make it easier for us to enter this "thin space" around the spirit, to borrow a concept from Celtic spirituality.[5] But we have to ask ourselves if we are brave enough to go there. What may we find? What does this mean?

Grief is common to care partnerships involving persons living with dementia or other chronic or terminal conditions.[6] We certainly grieve what we perceive as the loss of our care partner who is living with dementia. But also, I believe we grieve the loss of our own egoic (or mental) construct of the person and the nature of the relationship as it has been characterized historically and which is no longer operable due to dementia. Furthermore, we grieve the loss of our construct of our own self as it has existed in the relationship. It is crucial to remember that relationship still can occur, just not exactly like it has in the past.

It is unfair to hold someone who is living with dementia accountable to be what our egos desire them to be. Sure, we may continue to cherish the relationship as it has been in the past, but we must dare to let go of that image so that we will be free to have a relationship with our loved ones in their current state, realizing the core of personhood remains but must be honored in its ever-evolving representation. This will require flexibility and intentionality on the part of the care partner. And the freedom and compassion to let ourselves grieve.

But why bravery? Sometimes it may help care partners to deal with their own pain if they see their loved ones as no longer fully present. We may consider too painful the thought that our loved ones might be locked

---

4. Rohr, *Naked Now*, 122–23.
5. See "Thin Places."
6. Blandin and Pepin, "Dementia Grief," 67—78.

inside a mind that is racked by dementia, acutely suffering their losses that pile up daily. It may give us unconscious comfort to consider them less than they were, less able to feel and know and, therefore, to hurt. Such reductionism can be a protective mechanism for care partners and loved ones.

But if we can summon the courage to consider the core still present and to come alongside our loved ones again in spirit if we are not able to in body, though we may weep, our "weeping may unleash the fires of hope within us," as expressed so poignantly by Simone Campbell.[7] Facing truth in this way also brings us face to face with our own mortality, which all of us resist (even health care providers resist this, perhaps explaining why we providers often avoid painful conversations with our patients). But the truth must always come out, and when it does, we may find ourselves within the realm of the spiritual: mitigating our existential angst through accepting the inevitability of death and incorporating its essential threads into the fabric of our transcendent lives.

Many different spiritual traditions teach the importance of diminishment in the process of enlightenment. For instance, medieval mystic Meister Eckhart said, "God is not found . . . by adding anything, but by a process of subtraction."[8] Learning how to remove the accoutrements with which culture dresses us, we may thus be enabled to encounter each other's souls, including those who are living with dementia, unencumbered by the disease process. We must be willing to dwell in the present, for it is along the leading edge of the present moment where such encounters happen.

Centering ourselves on the selfhood of another in the unfolding present can be a self-emptying experience which has rewards that are paradoxically filling. Through this very spiritual act, we are able to enter into the lines of another person's story, to take up our part as an observer there. If conditions are right, we may briefly *become* the other by the embodiment wrought through empathy. This enfleshment of another life I consider to be the highest aspiration of the spiritual journey through dementia.

It is possible to consider the eye with which we are seeing the other person and their story as the same eye with which we ourselves are seen and known, even in our human "dis-ease." This is the vision of God which none of us in this life may ever hope to co-opt but through which we are given brief access—as much as we, in our frailty, are able to bear.

---

7. From notes taken at the 2015 CONSPIRE conference presented by the Center for Action and Contemplation on July 10–12, 2015.

8. Fox, *Meister Eckhart*, 41.

Part I: Prelude and Program Description

Having found ourselves in such a sacred space, how could we not bow in awe? The sheer face of the spirit, thus beheld, is grander than a mountain vista at sunrise. The expression of awe, gratitude, even worship is an innate response to such a beholding. So, we are led through the realm of the spiritual with courage, letting go, acceptance, weeping, listening, giving, focusing, seeing, staying, centering, transcending.

We are changed from encounters like these. Venturing into the depths, we come back different. We have treasures to show and stories to tell. We are witnesses-turned-evangelists. The light of the story then radiates from us. And this is key: *our own inner light is kindled by that of another, and we are able to share this light.* The communal light of many candles can light the world of dementia care, if we will let them burn.

I myself am in awe of the loving care I have seen expressed by so many care partners and the courageous living of persons with dementia. I do not dare try to instruct someone who has walked or who is walking this road. I also realize that the demands or experience of care partnering may make it very difficult to see anything redemptive about it, to consider the spiritual at all in the struggles. And I respect that. What I have written here is shared simply to encourage, to offer a paradigm that I and many others have found to be health and peace promoting, and to offer hope that I know is needed by those on this journey.

I acknowledge, in deep gratitude, all who have shared parts of their vision with me, and I hope that this framework will increase the transformational impact of Bringing Art to Life.

Part II

The Stories

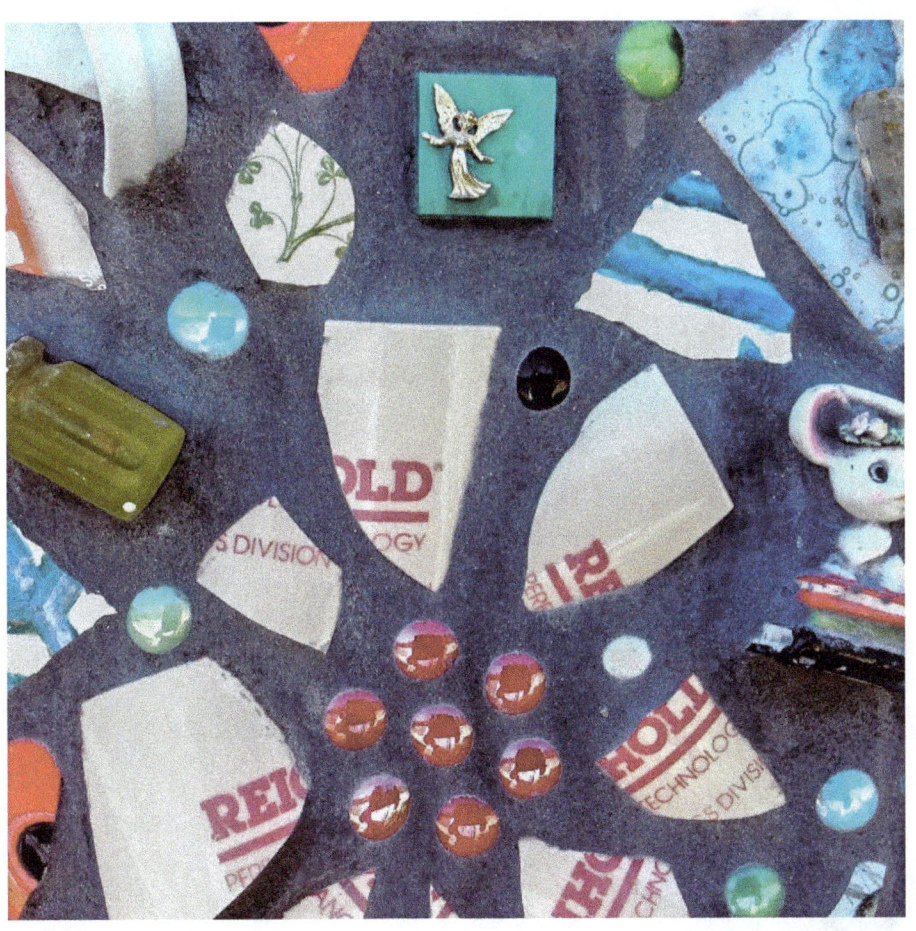

A Word about the Stories

> Stories have to be told or they die, and when they die, we can't remember who we are or why we're here.
>
> —SUE MONK KIDD

> To hell with facts! We need stories!
>
> —KEN KESEY

OUR BATL STUDENTS SOMETIMES get stressed when they feel they are not acquiring enough life-story material with which to build a legacy book for their dementia partners.

As the program evolved, we realized that we wanted the legacy books to be the students' artistic representation of their dementia partners' lives, a portrait of their personhood through students' eyes rather than a chronological, factual accounting. The latter would not be possible in this paradigm and might be an exercise in frustration. This method of offering a legacy book honors the creativity and imagination of the students and gives them an opportunity to add their own colors to the mixture, some of which may be slightly different shades after developing new friendships through the program.

In presenting stories for this book, I have adopted a similar philosophy. My method has been to flesh as much as I could from my own recollection of a particular session, then to build a story that is as true as possible

Part II: The Stories

to what I can remember of the impact of the event itself, the emotional tone and physical setting of the moment in which the event occurred, the personhood of those involved, and the relational structure in which the recollection is held. After setting this on paper as many times as possible, I have attempted to test and inform my memories by rereading student writings and my own and art therapist's notes, and by reaching out to former students for their current reflections on these past experiences.

I have taken the liberty of changing names, realizing that the content of each story inherently preserves the essence of each individual about whom the story is told. Some details have clearly been missed. But my hope is that much of the truth of each event from the time of its unfolding has been retained and retold herein.

It was a very difficult undertaking to choose which stories to highlight here. There are so many "Bringing Art to Life moments," as we call them. But I trust the untold stories somehow have provided steady companionship to the writer as he has written them, quietly affirming, nudgingly correcting, and knowingly editing with an unseen hand.

I tell these stories again so that some part of them, and of the characters in them, will always be remembered. I feel an obligation to share them, since I am the only person who has been there for all the sessions. And I hope something in them will resonate with you, the reader, as they have with me. Then, a time may come when we will remember them together. Is not memory rightly considered a communal concept? Perhaps relational remembering is the best treatment for our collective forgetting, against which we stand together in all the resiliency of human existence. As the Reverend Dr. Gary Furr, our friend and one of our BATL musicians, has beautifully said, "To be remembered and never forgotten is to continue being loved."

We live to claim our stories. With them, let us love each other and ourselves.

Maria and Madre

> People think of me differently because I'm Mexican.
> I try to show them that I am everything.
>
> —MARIA

THOSE WHO HAVE BEEN present during group art therapy sessions with persons who are living with dementia know that the collective creative act conducted within a safe and supportive space calls forth autobiographical memories—life-story elements that may have been submerged under many cognitive and social layers, floating in subterranean channels of neural connectivity.

When wading in a stream, we are apt to find many lovely things, and some things by which we may be bitten. But the call of the water is strong, and life is worth wading into together.

A neurologist, I was unfamiliar with the practice of art therapy until I met Angel Duncan, about whom I have spoken earlier in this book. Angel visited Tuscaloosa after learning of Dad's story, eventually assumed the role of executive arts director of Cognitive Dynamics, and helped us create BATL and our other programs. It was Angel who initially taught me some art therapy history, theory, methods, and directives, and shared stories from her extensive experience working with persons living with dementia in programs and institutions from coast to coast. Angel remains an integral part of BATL and has helped us recruit local art therapists to teach and facilitate in the program.

Part II: The Stories

The component of art therapy that has impressed me the most is the emotional processing that is facilitated by the therapist when memories come to the surface, be they joyful, humorous, anxiety-provoking, traumatic, sad, etc. Occasionally, our dementia partners will tap a discomforting memory, one that holds some emotional pain, and they may cry. But crying can be very therapeutic.

All of us, as we age, need opportunities to work through certain psychological wounds linked to traumatic experiences or unresolved conflicts earlier in life, which can be difficult even for those of us without cognitive impairment. With dementia thrown into the mix, the task of dealing with these issues could be daunting and is thought to be a common cause of challenging behaviors that often emerge in persons living with dementia (as they might in any of us).[1] Tragically, these behaviors too often result in the administration of pharmacological or, frankly, punitive interventions which may be harmful, when they should be seen as portals into the needs of persons living with dementia that are clamoring to be met.

The impact of observing the aforementioned processing has been profound, and there are too many narratives to share that would emphasize this point. None is more beautifully illustrative, however, than the story of Maria and her Madre.

Maria, a Hispanic woman of about seventy living with early-onset Alzheimer's disease, was a lively, beautiful, fiercely independent soul who held fast to her place in a strong line of matriarchal succession. The glory of her smile and her infectious laughter spread deftly over the room as she created her art and told stories of her formative years in sun-soaked Southwestern climes. But there was pain as well, hiding just beneath the surface. We saw it at times in a frightened look, an anxious movement, or a down-turned face; we heard it quivering in her voice.

Maria had mentioned her mother ("Madre") on a few occasions, and the students had pieced enough of the story together to know something of her affection. But there was an untouched sadness that cried out for healing, as evidenced by this interchange between Maria and our art therapist, Karen Gibbons, over a piece of art she had created:

"Does this artwork bring anything particular to mind for you, Maria?"

"My mother."

"How do you feel when you think about your mother and your artwork?"

---

1. Feil, *Validation Breakthrough*, 3–7.

Maria and Madre

"Sad."

"If it makes you feel sad, how do you turn that to a happy feeling?"

"I talk to her."

In her book *The Validation Breakthrough*, pioneering dementia caregiving teacher Naomi Feil speaks about a commonly observed phenomenon in older adults living with cognitive impairment: speaking with or continuing to maintain relationships with loved ones who are deceased as a means of meeting certain psychological needs.[2] It appeared that Maria needed to meet with Madre (perhaps Madre also needed to meet with Maria).

In the following week's session, the directive Karen selected was finger painting Japanese paper lanterns with acrylic paints. I remember that Maria came in acting differently that day: not as interactive, smiling less, and laughing little. During the description of the art therapy directive, she seemed troubled and ill-attentive. I wondered if the sentiments she had expressed the week prior were evidence that some hidden door, closed long ago, was beginning to crack open. A door to a room full of unresolved guilt, grief, sadness, perhaps even anger. But who could know for sure? I had hoped the directive would help. But then she entered in such a state.

The students helped to get her paints ready as she donned a rubber glove on each hand. Hesitantly, Maria picked out her paint color: a deep cobalt blue. As the students squeezed out a blue blob onto her fingers, Maria started speaking about Madre, focusing on how she had cared for her during a chronic illness and of how the attending physicians never told her how her mother finally had died. We assumed, upon hearing this, that Maria may not have been present at the time of her mother's death and could have been remorseful.

Over the years, some of the details of the session have faded from my memory. But the tone Maria emoted is indelible. Even now, I can feel the pain imbedded in this tale of a daughter and her mother, of the deep caring and compassion she must have shared in those days prior to departure, and of the desire to take again her Madre into a long and loving embrace.

Then, something began to happen. I am not able to say exactly when the atmosphere in the room started to change, caught up as I was by the turning of the lantern in her fingers, which were smeared with cobalt hues. Maria's countenance morphed from an expression of sadness to one of serenity, of contentment, of peace. As she tenderly anointed the lantern in blue, she spoke of how much she loved her mother and of wanting to tell

---

2. Feil, *Validation Breakthrough*, 3–7.

her so. The room became still and silent in her countenance, spellbound. The lantern had slowly turned. Turned. Turned. To blue. The tender blue longings of a mother's face.

When the entire surface had been covered and Maria had paused to simply look at her art, Karen posed the question, "Maria, what would you like to name your lantern?"

"Madre," she whispered, peaceably, like a mother to her newborn babe. "*Madre.*"

A Day Like Today

"What's your favorite holiday, Mr. Donny?"
"A day like today."
—BATL STUDENTS AND MR. DONNY

HE WAS SOLID. ONE look at Mr. Donny and you knew this about him. He was solid from way down deep, in the same way that my father had been.

First, he was an imposing physical specimen—strong, sturdy, more youthful than his seventy-six years might have allowed, with stove-pipe arms and beech-trunk thighs. He looked like something that had been rooted for decades in a West Alabama river bottom, like a Tombigbee tupelo or a Sipsey bald cypress; deeply set, firm, and silent, calmly surveying the meandering course of the blue-black water.

Later, we learned he had a solid work ethic as well and had designed and built his family a home with his own hands, and that he had assisted each of his children in doing the same for their families.

His faith and sense of service were as solid as his frame. Mr. Donny was a selfless giver, always looking for opportunities, and others, to help out. And he did so humbly, with no hoopla.

In BATL, we found him to be solidly rooted in the present moment, perhaps more so than any of our other participants had seemed to be. And he had a gift for helping those around him find their centers there as well.

As mentioned previously, the theory and practice of mindfulness form an important part of the core curriculum of BATL for several reasons. First, we feel it is essential to center oneself—mind, body, and spirit—in the present moment so that conditions will be right to experience deep relationships of the type we hope to cultivate with our dementia partners and amongst ourselves. Additionally, nonjudgmental, non-egoic acceptance of the reality one meets in the now is important. This is especially true for the *person* one meets there.

We should have no preconceived ideas about our dementia partners, their limitations or losses, their gifts, what they will be capable of accomplishing in art therapy, etc. This does not mean that we should not acquire knowledge about their dementia-associated deficits and identify ways that we may need to modify our communication strategies to be most effective, or that we should not guard against structuring art activities in ways that might inadvertently magnify their struggles or challenges. But it does mean that we should be completely present to, accepting of, and grateful for whomever we find sitting right in front of us in dementia's disguise.

Working through such a framework, one is more apt to develop a non-dual, or contemplative, way of seeing and experiencing reality as it is without being tempted to split its gray shades into black or white. One may be more likely to cultivate the gratitude that naturally germinates in such an open, accepting, unitive space. "Contemplation has been well-described as a long, loving look at the Real," says Franciscan priest and author Father Richard Rohr—as celebrating the "sacrament of the present moment," and of "finding God in what is right in front of you."[1] Such a view can give one a sense of awe even in the common or mundane, as well as the proclivity to seek the depths in those with whom one is in relationship, thereby also accessing the deeper parts of oneself.

Mr. Donny seemed to possess this contemplative way of seeing, of being present, and of reaching in to take hold of the joy that is possible to claim within, regardless of the circumstances in which we find ourselves. And he routinely shared this joy with all of us in BATL.

At first, we wondered if Mr. Donny would appreciate art making, but we soon had our concerns alleviated, as he delved headlong into the directives. Thinking we had him pegged after the first two sessions as someone whose lines always were straight, whose shapes were squared off and stacked, and who painted only within the margins, we were surprised to see the abandon with which he approached the shoebox art, placing any object he could find onto the paint globs before shaking and agitating recklessly.

---

1. Rohr, *Just This*, 29.

"Some of it's good, and some of it's not," he would say of his art, prompting the students to see the deeper significance of his statement. Some days were good, and some were not. But Donny seemed to be able to find the good in all of them, to find something about which to be joyful. Indeed, every day—including its experiences, relationships, shared space, and shared activities—appeared to be special to Mr. Donny. Being around this man changed the lives of several of our students, and they wrote about this transformation:

> You always have a smile on your face, and you always naturally see the good in every situation. Thank you for brightening all my days with your positivity and enthusiasm. Thank you for teaching me to overcome any obstacles that life throws at me, and thank you for allowing me to spend time with you.

> You have taught me so much about joy, patience, and authentic relationships. I have seen you choose joy when you are anxious. I have seen you persevere when things are hard. You have given me a fresh perspective on what it means to really listen to and know someone. Your life has left a huge mark on mine, one that I'm so grateful for.

Our late-October, fall-themed art therapy directive involved decorating pumpkins: one could choose whether to paint them and what color, and there were many objects that could be glued or painted onto them as well. Mr. Donny chose to brush his meticulously in black, after which he glued on a set of pink lips, a couple of whimsical ghosts, and a richly tinted leaf, the latter signifying his love of and appreciation for nature, which his family had commented was well known.

After Mr. Donny had finished his pumpkin, the art therapist commented on how much art he had created that day, and, being a man of few words, Mr. Donny replied, "Yep," then clapped for himself. Everyone joined in, and we all had a good laugh about it. But he really did appear to be proud of his accomplishments, just as my father had been about his artistic creations.

Before the session ended, one of his students asked Mr. Donny to tell us his favorite holiday. To which he replied, with a look of contentment, peace, and belonging in his eyes, "A day like today." This became the quote of the semester and has remained one of the quotes I share with each crop of new students as I'm explaining what they can expect in their BATL experience.

Part II: The Stories

Mr. Donny was living with mixed dementia, Alzheimer's plus vascular. He no longer could drive, hold a job, or build things for others like he used to. He had trouble getting his words out, couldn't remember most of his family members' names, had to have help going to the bathroom and getting dressed, and was able to say only a few words in choppy sentences. Yet, in his dementia-tainted reality, he was able to regard an ordinary day to be just as special as his favorite holiday. We all hoped we had played some part in making that day special for him.

We hoped also that because of Donny, we would be able to find a pair of prankster pink lips, some fiery fall leaves, and a couple of quirky little ghosts with which to adorn even our darkest days to come.

Helping Miss Carrie

> Thank you for thinking of me.
> —MISS CARRIE

MISS CARRIE WAS KNOWN in the community as a helper, especially of struggling young people. With her head, her heart, and her hands, she cared for folks and families and helped to put their lives back together. She was a poignant painting of a kind and humble servant.

"The Lord has blessed us with these things, so we need to show others God's love," she would say.

Miss Carrie continued to be active in the community and in her church until advancing Parkinson's disease, with its associated dementia, rendered her more dependent, and she enrolled at Caring Days.

Something gentle and serene rose up out of Miss Carrie and touched us all. Her students sat rapt beside her during art therapy. I watched, too, and pondered.

During one particular session, the activity involved, again, shoebox art (This activity, you may have guessed, is one of our favorites). Clients chose colors of paint to drop onto the floor of a shoebox, then added some marbles and other available items, such as feathers. The box was then closed and shaken, spreading the paint randomly in wildly unique color patterns.

The activity appeared to interest Miss Carrie, but I suspect all of us were thinking the same thing. With her parkinsonian tremor, stiffness, and loss of motor control, would she be able to fully participate? Would the activity be a meaningful one for her? Would it be an exercise in frustration or, God forbid, a source of embarrassment for her?

One of the phenomena that develops in BATL is the organic nature of the small-group dynamic as it morphs into a circle dance of relationships. Each group becomes, by the end of the semester, a single interdependent entity within the larger group-whole, rather than separate individuals merely taking their places in proximity to each other. The winds of this deep and growing connection both drive behavior and are attested to by the response of each group member, as the ebb and sway of loblolly pines lend evidence of an invisible bayside breeze.

The magic began to happen as Miss Carrie reached for a bottle of paint. Realizing she would be challenged by this task, she asked one of her students if she would grasp the paint bottle and let Miss Carrie simply take hold of her wrist, guiding the student's hand to the spots where she wanted to place the paint drops. The students affirmed this idea, and the new care partnership began to take shape.

After a few blobs of paint were successfully placed, Miss Carrie asked if she herself could reach for the marbles with the students' help. Everyone agreed that this would be a good idea. Miss Carrie then took a marble into her grasp, steadied by the hands of her students, and placed it into a paint blob in the shoebox. Then another and another. Followed by a few feathers. Then the shoebox was sealed.

She grinned as she took the box and began to agitate it. Her whole body moved in the rhythms that she determined to follow. No one helped her to do this; at least, not physically. But all of us were silently cheering her on in the beautiful dance of creativity that was playing out before us. And it seemed her Parkinson's disease sat this one out.

At last, the box top was removed to show the unpredicted beauty of her art, shaken, stirred, stilled. She seemed so proud of it and showed it to the whole group. Then followed some of her story that had been in hiding for a long time, pouring forth into the open hands of the moment. The students listened and learned of her humanity, of her people, of her home, and of her God.

As time ran out on the session, Miss Carrie offered this expression of gratitude to all of us: "Thank you for thinking of me."

A few weeks later, at our final celebratory dinner, her students got up and shared how much Miss Carrie had impacted their lives, setting her family members abeam with pride. After the students had presented her art

Helping Miss Carrie

and legacy book, Miss Carrie got up and gave an impromptu speech to the crowd. Though she said many of the things she had shared in the previous weeks, the artist of the present moment painted her words ever new.

We heard from Miss Carrie's family a few months later. After the BATL experience that fall, Miss Carrie apparently had been much more present and interactive during family gatherings over the holidays, and many pleasant memories had been created. They then shared that Miss Carrie had recently passed away and how much it had meant to them to have had those days with her, those days after BATL, and of how they cherished the celebratory dinner experience.

Miss Carrie's students have moved on down their life paths now and are young physicians bearing through the rigors of residency training. Every few months I will hear from them, and we remember our BATL moments together. Sometimes, out of the blue, I'll email them a photo of their hands helping Miss Carrie, to remind them of who they are and what they've been called to do.

Ernie's Hands

He's got you and me, brother, in His hands,
He's got you and me, sister, in His hands,
He's got everybody in His hands,
He's got the whole world in His hands.[1]

—AFRICAN AMERICAN SPIRITUAL

HE WALKED TO THE store one night to get groceries for his mother. Someone attacked him and left him for dead. In truth, he was very close to it.

For the next several weeks, Ernie lay in an intensive care unit on life support, comatose, with little hope of recovery. The doctors made their rounds and prognostications. But with every passing day, it became less likely that Ernie would wake up or have any prospect of meaningful neurological recovery.

Though he was in a coma, Ernie heard the doctors speaking about fading hope. He remembered the grim tone of their voices, their gray, expressionless faces. The room looked like a shadow to him. But he could see himself lying there, lifeless. He saw the medical team exit, leaving him and his mother alone. He heard her softly praying for him. Telling him

---

[1]. Shortly before Jessye Norman died, a friend of mine was in attendance when she made an appearance at Ponce de Leon Baptist Church in Atlanta to sing her signature "He's Got the Whole World in His Hands." Although elderly and confined to a motorized wheelchair, she sang it as well as ever. Her singing of that song despite age and disability is a good example of the concept of pillars of personhood.

everything would be all right. Assuring him she would take care of him. That she would never give up on him. That she would always pray for him.

One day, Ernie woke up. The doctors were baffled. Mother was not. She was only grateful, thanking God for answered prayer.

After prolonged inpatient rehabilitation, Ernie was able to return home to his mother, who essentially became his sole caregiver. Ernie's dog, a chihuahua, was waiting on him when he arrived.

He loved this little dog. He loved his mother. And, as we would one day discover, he loved everything and everyone else.

Ernie, at fifty-four, was one of the younger clients at Caring Days, but one of the most debilitated. Because he was partially paralyzed, his left hand and arm were drawn into flexion, and he had little use of that side. He leaned forward from the waste at quite an acute angle and shuffled behind a walker at a slow pace. But his smile and joyous spirit preceded him into every room, into every encounter with friends, new and old.

Ernie was the first person with traumatic brain injury who was selected to participate in BATL, and this gave us an opportunity to broaden out our educational offerings in preparation for the first art therapy session, when Ernie would meet his group of student partners. The traumatic injury had damaged multiple regions of Ernie's brain, affecting his speech and language, memory, and other aspects of his cognition, in addition to his motor function and balance. There also was some disinhibition, which promoted freedom of emotional expression that was to enliven our ensuing art therapy sessions and paint the room in the vibrant and loving colors of Ernie's heart.

We soon learned of Ernie's love and appreciation for his mother and of how much he trusted her. "My Mama always takes care of me," he said many times. "I like to watch her in the garden taking care of her flowers too." He would sit on the porch and observe his mother's tending of the plants.

Ernie displayed a trait that we have witnessed over and over in our BATL partners. He often mentioned sadness, loss, or struggle. But he always followed this with messages of hope. For example, he related the story above, about seeing the hospital room, finishing this recount with the prayer of his mother. "I love my little dog," he would say, "but I know he will die someday. My Mama is eighty-one. She takes care of me. I don't want her to die." For a moment, he seemed to turn inward, the joyful facial expression briefly turning pensive. Then, as if suddenly seeing his mother in the garden again, he would smile and tell a story about her.

Part II: The Stories

One of our favorite art therapy directives is an exercise in which the hands are traced onto paper in the color of one's choice, then participants are encouraged to add words or images of what their hands have done, some of their favorite things, important content of their lives or stories, hobbies, or other elements of their personhood. The students often end up helping their participants with the hand tracing and adding of elements, especially if there is a physical handicap affecting the use of the hands. Thinking back on several years of observing this activity, I am deeply moved to recall the hands of students and their dementia partners, young and old juxtaposed, often with different skin colors, mingling together in art making, coming to know and trust each other in these vulnerable moments of human expression.

When it came time to trace Ernie's hands, I wondered about the paralyzed left side and if he wouldn't want that hand traced. Without any hesitancy, he placed both hands on the paper and asked the students to begin tracing. Something beautiful happened as the contrasting shapes of the two hands appeared on the page, one finger of the contracted hand pointing toward the right, anointed with the dark outline of a student's marker.

Ernie then selected markers of his own and began to talk about things he loved as he added them to his artwork. We were amazed to see that he added some of his favorite things to the image of the paralyzed hand: a saxophone, a TV, and a frisbee, signifying his favorite pastimes. Then the figure of a person began to take shape on some of the fingers that had been drawn into flexion by the wounded neurons injured in the hateful act that had nearly ended his life. It was the shape of a person. "This is my Mama. My Mama takes care of me. I love my Mama," he witnessed to all of us.

It looked to me like Mama had come to bring healing to the hand of her beloved son.

A few weeks later, in the final art therapy session, participants were asked to paint a self-portrait made of watercolors. For his portrait, Ernie painted a crimson heart (Ernie also loved Alabama football and spoke often of his heroes on the team), and when it dried, a glowing golden sun superimposed. "Life is beautiful," he told all of us, "and I'm happy to be here with all of you."

We will always be happy, too, when we think of Ernie, his Mama, and his hands.

After our time with Ernie had come to a close, I wondered what would have happened if Ernie's attackers had been present with us during art therapy. What Ernie might have said to them. What color he might have painted them. Then, I realized that they had been there, right in the room, in the subconscious recesses of Ernie's mind, where his mother prayed as she tended the plants in her garden. And he had drawn them in vanishing ink on the skin of his wounded hand.

A Smile and a Handshake

> A smile and a handshake don't cost a dime.
>
> —MISS DORIS

MANY THINGS ABOUT MISS DORIS and our time with her are etched in my memory. I had known her husband before I met her. He was one of the first patients I saw upon beginning my new neurology practice in 1997. He reminded me quite a lot of my dad—cut of the same canvas, so to speak. About the time I was diagnosing Miss Doris's husband with Parkinson's disease, Dad was showing early signs of Alzheimer's that I did not recognize (or perhaps denied). Why does familial relationship often blind us to reality?

Through Miss Doris's husband, I met other family members, and their two daughters became friends of mine over the years. Truthfully, I love the family. It would be hard not to. And this had absolutely nothing to do with fudge. Then again, that may not entirely be true.

My first contact with Miss Doris came around the holidays after her husband had passed away. She brought some chocolate fudge by the office for the staff and me, and I happened to be out of town that week. Fortunately, a nurse saved some for me, as most of that batch was eaten by others. I don't hold it against them. It was mighty fine fudge, as many folks in the community could attest. But as delectable as it was, this is not my strongest memory of Miss Doris.

Looking back over the years of medical practice, I can recall many cases in which the caregiver for a certain patient living with a chronic neurological illness eventually became my patient as well. I have found no connections with particular diagnoses, just that caregivers appear to develop chronic illnesses of their own at a disproportionately higher rate. Research bears this out. According to the Family Caregiving Alliance, studies consistently show higher levels of depressive symptoms and mental health problems among caregivers than their non-caregiving peers, and nearly twice the rate of chronic health conditions is reported.[1]

Initially, Miss Doris sought my care for numbness in a hand. However, it became apparent through my own observations and reports from her family that cognitive dysfunction was beginning to manifest itself. Eventually, a diagnosis of Alzheimer's was made. In my opinion, it is particularly difficult to witness the ravages of dementia upon those who have been so independent, self-sufficient, and benevolent as Miss Doris—individuals in whose personhood whole families and even communities are held together. Roles change, some organically, some as the result of interventions that are met with resistance. None without some kind of pain or wounding to the psyche and spirit. The impact of making a diagnosis of dementia is always profound for me, and I remember many of the emotions I felt in this case. But this is not my strongest memory of Miss Doris.

The time came when this capable woman no longer could care for herself at home, and her family enrolled her as a client at Caring Days. Shortly afterward, she became a participant in BATL, for which I was thankful. Her students, and all of us, learned so much from her about how life should be lived. About raising a banner of courage in the fields of adversity, about building bridges of generativity in the waters of stagnation. About caring for the young hearts entrusted to us, both of others and of ourselves.

Greetings tended to be the same in each art therapy session with Miss Doris, and that was alright by us. "A smile and a handshake don't cost a dime," she would always say, demonstrating both to the students, who received them like it was the first time they'd been offered.

Miss Doris's tone tended to change a bit after the art therapy directive for the day had been presented. "I'm not an artist," she would retort, to which the art therapist offered an invitation to try something new with the students. She tended, like some others, to assume the role of a teacher or mentor on those occasions, asking the students what they wanted to make, taking delight in anything they desired to show her. That was the kind of interaction in which she seemed to feel most comfortable, and we learned

---

1. Pinquart and Sorensen, "Caregivers and Noncaregivers," 250–67.

that what we were seeing at those times was the inner Doris coming out in all her selfsame glory.

She often spoke of the time she and her husband spent as youth leaders of their local church and of how the door always had been open to the young people, who knew their home to be a sanctuary of acceptance and belonging. A safe haven in times of seeking. Love abided there, and apparently, the youth of their community knew it. And this grace extended out beyond their own congregation. Some who had been impacted by such a presence in their formative years remained lifelong friends of Miss Doris and her husband, visiting them again over the years. I understand there were many late nights in their household—conversations, confessions, prayers, and pardons, where the welcome knew no curfew.

"Have I seen you before?" she tended to say each week to one premed student in her small group. He looked a bit like me in younger days, and I couldn't help but wonder if a characteristic of our faces had jump-started some of her idling neurons.

I find myself hoping that same thing in most of my interactions. Not the angle of my nose, or that scar on my forehead from a nearly sightless childhood encounter with my grandfather's pocketknife, or the way one of my ears is slightly lower than the other, or the mark on my temple from the forceps at birth, or even the spectacles that make me look smarter than I am. Nothing like that. But something in my eyes that seems to be singing their song back to them after they've forgotten it, a movement of my mouth that springs forth medicinal draught for which their bodies are aching, or an entry to some sanctuary for the lonely, frightened child through which they might stumble at the threshold of my smile.

None of these are saintly traits that I've recognized and developed intentionally, for which I've piously offered prayers of thanksgiving. Rather, these are sproutings from the leading edges of wounds in my own soul; some self-inflicted, upon which the balm of grace has been applied; grace to fill the gaps. Will these healing wounds be charged with energy enough to cross synaptic connections that allow my face to communicate with theirs? With hers? I pray so.

She spoke about making baby blankets and how she enjoyed doing it. I seem to remember she had done this for all the children in her family. Some months later, through tears, her daughter told us that Miss Doris had not been able to finish the last one. But this is not my strongest memory of Miss Doris.

A Smile and a Handshake

What I remember the most about Miss Doris is the impact her life made on others. The affections she kindled in people, young and old, whom she had touched with her kindness, her humor, her strength. I remember the students as they stood, one by one, at the end-of-semester BATL celebratory dinner and told how much she meant to them, how much they appreciated the wisdom she had shared, how grateful they were for her willingness to make art with them and tell them stories of her life. And of how much they thanked her for caring about young people. And I remember the heartfelt video her family made to honor her. We played it that night. What a legacy. What a life! That's what I remember most about Miss Doris.

"A smile and a handshake don't cost a dime."

I wish I could hear her say that again in person. This time, I'd pay her back with a heart full of gold for my neighbors and an always-open door.

He Taught Us How to Listen

There's a lot of difference between listening and hearing.
—G. K. CHESTERTON

IN THE NEWSPAPER SOME time ago, I read of the passing of a good man, Roy, one of our former BATL participants.

Roy was well respected and accomplished and had done a lifetime of good work. He was intelligent and proficient, we had learned, and had once built a functional computer, a feat about which the technologically challenged, like me, were in awe. A healthcare administrator by profession, Roy had made a career of, among other things, devising and implementing solutions to communication problems, creating pathways of greater efficiency in the acquisition, storage, retrieval, and transfer of information. You might say he'd been building, of a sort, bionic brains for broken bodies.

With this background, perhaps one can better appreciate the particular cruelty of Alzheimer's, which was breaking Roy's brain into a clump of impotent, cross-wired, misfiring entanglements.

We felt it would be somewhat of a challenge to create a meaningful experience for Roy and for the students working with him, given his language impairments. As part of the educational content of the program, we cover mindful listening techniques and emphasize the importance of cultivating patience and compassionate, unshifting, non-distracting, non-egoic attention to every element of expression employed by persons living with dementia to get their message across. We teach the assumption of a proper posture by the listener, a gentle "leaning into" the story of the other to perceive the faintest whisper of the self without attempting to pull anything out of them, creating and defending a safe and silent space into which verbal and nonverbal communication may flow, may be received, and may be validated.

We need not know what we think we need to know. Instead, we need to know what we are needed to know. (Please read that again.) This is selfless and tender work, indeed, and is not easy for anyone. A sacred occupation, I would assert. And essential for the program to be effective for persons like Roy, and for our students.

More than any of the others we had that semester, the interaction with Roy was an emotional one for me because his language problems reminded me of Dad's, hitting close to home. I found myself feeling so much compassion for him when he was in the middle of phrases and trying so hard to get the words out. It amazed me that, even after long pauses, he was still able to maintain his thought and focus enough to complete his sentences if given enough space, time, and attention.

One day while we were near him and listening, he managed to get out a story that was very important to him—obviously something he needed us to hear. It was a story about a meaningful time in his life when he had done a selfless act for his colleagues. There had been a severe snowstorm, and he had organized and participated in a rescue mission for some of his coworkers. It took several minutes for him get the story out, piecemeal, but the more words and thoughts expressed, the richer and deeper the impact of the story on all of us. And the more of himself we observed. There Roy was, coming to the rescue of his own personhood, which lay trapped in the winter storm of Alzheimer's. We followed him there.

As mentioned previously, cognitive impairment may be particularly distressing for persons living with dementia who have come to prize and rely upon their intellect over other traits (and caregivers for whom the intellectual component of their loved one's personhood is most revered, or upon which the family dynamic has been built). I suspect this was true of Roy, and it might have tended to make him feel "less than" in his losses. But I am so proud of his three student partners for the empathy, compassion, and patience they showed him, truly validating Roy in the reality of his present moment experience.

Roy's disease was the most advanced of the group that semester, and his language disturbance and executive problems were the most severe.

Part II: The Stories

When our musical guests Shades Mountain Air[1] sang a moving number called "Words Fail" during one of our art therapy sessions, I became emotional thinking of Roy. In contrast, the actions of love and compassion directed toward Roy by his student partners did not fail to give him the honor and dignity he deserved.

Another touching story about Roy involved someone in his circle of friends and care partners and was told to the students by Roy's family during the assembly of his life-legacy book. Roy and his wife and some friends shared a love of choral singing, and after Roy's impairment made it difficult for him to participate, his supporters collaborated to help him get robed, find his music, and stay engaged during the worship service. So that the process of helping Roy to robe would not highlight his lack of independence or his growing infirmities, Roy's designated robing helper asked someone to assist him with his own robe as well. Apparently, this gesture sparked others to do the same, so that those choir members near Roy helped each other robe up each week. I find this to be a beautiful example of creating a culture of compassion in dementia care.

When he told his tale of a daring rescue in the snow, Roy taught us how to listen—intently, mindfully, compassionately—and he taught us about the rewards to be found if we do. He showed so much courage in sharing his story at a time when many might have chosen to be silent out of frustration, fear, or shame. And the students sat quietly at attention out of honor and respect. And out of a desire to bring their best to the high calling of such an experience. What Roy shared was a glimpse into the content of his character. And Alzheimer's hadn't stolen that. Could not. *Cannot*, in fact.

Thank you, Roy, brave and storied soul, for venturing out into the snow with your self to rescue us all. We hear you calling. And we promise to go on listening.

Requiescat in pace.

---

1. You can listen to Shades Mountain Air on Spotify.

Some Things Are Meant to Be

If only you could sense how important you are to the lives of those you meet; how important you can be to people you may never even dream of. There is something of yourself that you leave at every meeting with another person.

—FRED ROGERS

I ALWAYS LOOK FORWARD, somewhat nervously, to the first art therapy session of each semester. This is when the magic starts to spark.

As usual, our first directive one particular semester was a collage activity in which participants use magazine images and stickers as a means of introducing themselves to the group. The chosen images often represent family, occupation, interests, hobbies, friends, pets, etc. According to Dr. Carrie Ezelle, one of our BATL art therapists, this directive is a "non-threatening introduction to art making and provides comfortable distance for expression that is ideal for an early session's goals of getting to know participants and the group." The activity acclimates everyone to creative expression and highlights some important self elements that may be looking for an outlet. Stress usually lessens through this directive, and "clients may experience increased self-esteem and self-worth."[1]

A pair of female students had met their participant one week before. Janice, a woman in her early seventies with moderately advanced Alzheimer's, was slender, petite, gentle in her movements, and somewhat shy except when it came to hugs. She was widely recognized as the best hugger at Caring Days. Janice tended to get a bit agitated at times thinking she would

---

1. Dr. Carrie Ezelle, email message to author, January 6, 2017.

miss her husband when he came to pick her up, and staff had found hugs to be the only restraints that were needed. This method had never failed to tip over the spinning top of anxiety and reset the moment in an atmosphere of comfort. Except for that day.

Janice's students placed some magazines and stickers on the table in front of her and asked what she wanted to look at. Images that she seemed to be interested in were then cut out and arranged for her to make selections for her collage. She was somewhat hesitant at times, but her students showed maturity, sensitivity, and compassion in fanning the flicker of her intentions. Janice eventually selected photos of nail polish, Ginger Rogers and Fred Astaire dancing together, guitars, forest areas for hunting, some kind of pie, etc. Janice appeared to connect with the art and especially seemed drawn to the nail polish photo, commenting that her husband had been trying to get her to paint her fingernails and that the colors in the photo had given her an idea of which to choose.

She selected purple and seemed to gravitate toward that color the whole semester. Purple has a rich history of significance, lying between the mystery and emotion of red and the dreams and vast emptiness of blue. "It is the badge of noble youth," wrote ancient Roman author Pliny. "It brightens every garment, and shares with gold the glory of the triumph."[2] Purple signifies dignity and devotion and was commonly worn during times of mourning by women in the nineteenth century. Its violet hues moved Édouard Manet to tell his friends that he had finally discovered the true color of the atmosphere: "Fresh air is violet. Three years from now, the whole world will work in violet."[3] "I think it pisses God off if you walk by the color purple in a field somewhere and don't notice it," writes Alice Walker in *The Color Purple*.[4] Perhaps these are some of the reasons why purple was chosen as the official color of the Alzheimer's awareness movement.[5] The Alzheimer's Association states the following on its website: "Purple is our signature color, combining the calm stability of blue and the passionate energy of red. Purple makes a statement about our Association and our supporters: we are strong and unrelenting in the fight against Alzheimer's disease."[6]

2. St. Claire, *Secret Lives of Color*, 159.

3. St. Claire, *Secret Lives of Color*, 173–74.

4. Walker, *Color Purple*, 195.

5. For a discussion about the official color of the Alzheimer's awareness movement, see "Our Story."

6. "Our Story," para. 7.

Some Things Are Meant to Be

Toward the end of the session, Janice began to lose focus on the art and started to look anxiously about the room. The students, art therapist, and I gently redirected her, but these efforts seemed minimally effective. She stood up and headed toward the window facing the front parking lot, and said, "I wonder where my husband is? Has he forgotten me? It's time to go home." She then moved back to her seat at the request of her students and briefly became reengaged in the art. But I could see her getting a distant look and decided to make my way beside her.

I knelt down on one knee and began to affirm her. The students, therapist, and I talked about her collage and listened. She said, again, that she was worried she would miss her husband when he came for her. Deep within, I saw something that moved me greatly. It was a panicked look that I interpreted as a fear of abandonment, another of the many lies of dementia scrolling like some terrible headline before her eyes, even in the midst of people who cared, who would do everything they could to supply comfort, compassion, and a sense of safety—even though she knew her husband loved her and would never leave her to be alone. Nothing we were saying was seeming to reach a place that could soothe her fears. Then something struck me to sing.

Over the years, we have developed a playlist of musical selections for BATL that often accompanies our art therapy sessions. We hadn't had the music on this particular day. I began to think through the selections, and one favorite that came to mind was "Can't Help Falling in Love," a song by Peretti, Creatore, and Weiss, made famous by Elvis Presley in the early 1960s.[7] I started in on the first few bars, and one of the students Googled the lyrics and helped me out. In a few seconds, the whole room became a mixture of soft humming with a few words mixed in: "Fools rush in . . . shall I stay . . . Hmmm . . . like a river . . . some things are meant to be . . . Hmmm."

What happened next instantly became a "Bringing Art to Life moment," as we like to call them . . . times of intense, transcendent relationality in which the power of dementia to define someone's life asymptotically approaches zero and a quality of pure presence exponentially approaches a state of utter unity of being.

Janice took her gaze off of the window and moved it around the room, into the faces of all those present, each a shade of purple in a living collage of smiles and hums and words directed toward her dignity and well-being. She

---

7. Wikipedia, s.v. "Can't Help Falling in Love," https://en.wikipedia.org/wiki/Can%27t_Help_Falling_in_Love.

Part II: The Stories

looked, lastly, to me as I knelt next to her at eye level. She then reached out, took my face in her hands, and, searching my eyes with intention and sincerity, said words that I couldn't interpret phonetically but felt I understood spiritually. As she did this, her countenance changed, becoming deeply expressive of tenderness, serenity, and compassion. The room sat spellbound, its air suspended in mystery and awe, as Janice held onto my face.

At this point, I think I stopped singing, as I wasn't sure what would come next. Would she try to kiss me? How would I respond? Could I use this as a teachable moment of empathy for the students and yet ensure proper maintenance of personal space and boundaries, to which all of us are entitled? After a few more seconds, as the song was nearing completion, Janice turned back to her collage, gaining interest again in arranging her selections and gluing them to the paper background. All of us started to breathe again, as if we had just seen, for the first time in our lives, the soft purples and golds of a sunrise cresting the peaks of the Grand Tetons.

After the session was completed and we had escorted Janice and the other clients to lunch, we processed what we had witnessed. I am always impressed at the students' perceptions and thoughts, and especially about how these experiences have affected them. We are changed by deep personal encounters like the one with Janice. I am convinced that therein lies the primary educational value of BATL. Reflecting on the profundity of what had happened, I wrote an email to the students that contained the following content:

> When we intentionally develop relationships with people who are living with dementia, we are changed. Learning to know them in their full personhood despite dementia's diminishment, we see that the qualities of selfhood lie too deep to be affected by a physical illness. We know a vibrancy of spirit pulsing beneath surface disability, and we build an environment of validation and trust so that this spirit will find channels of expression through shared present moment experiences within the integrity of the relationship, like the one we had experienced with Janice.
>
> We begin to see ourselves in this other person—perhaps even as this other one—our common frailties and challenges, as well as our gifts, triumphs and potential. Empathy calls forth our deep humanity. As we create supportive space for this other one to find her voice and sing, to find her muse and paint, so we set our own inner self to singing and painting, authenticity begetting authenticity, stigma and shame being replaced by acceptance and compassion. This, then, can become a template for other relationships.

Some Things Are Meant to Be

If we come seeking to make contact, we must believe personhood persists despite cognitive deficits. Lives are not defined by diagnoses. Persons living with cognitive impairment are not empty shells drained of the content of their humanity.

Realizing that the ability to communicate effectively with words may have been lost, we must hone our multi-sensory listening skills and heighten awareness of non-verbal cues, aligning ourselves to receive and respond appropriately to these messages. Non-verbal cues may carry emotional content; we should acknowledge and validate this content in our responses . . . [I praised them on the fine example I had seen of this in the recent art therapy session.]

Our stance should be one of openness, vulnerability, authenticity and non-judgement, and we should expect to find a human being in front of us who has a story that needs to be appreciated. This story, with its history, its present, and yes, its future, is laid out before us in the form of one who needs us to bring our best selves home to the interaction.

The language of kindness, gentleness, presence, mindfulness, silence, and peace will speak when words fail. Non-threatening touch, being mindful of response, can effectively communicate warmth and good intention. Resisting reactivity, we should validate the emotional content of their expression, but refrain from mirroring anxiety or agitation, instead using smiles, gentle eye contact, soft singing or humming, or props to create a non-threatening environment. The session with Janice was a living example of this approach. In particular, humming and singing a familiar tune had set the stage for the powerful moment with Janice . . . [Later, we were to find out that the song we sang to Janice—or, perhaps, that sang itself to her—held special meaning for her and her family].

We must quieten the hypercognitive chatter of the world in which we live, seeking instead a state of wakeful stillness and present moment centeredness, opening the all-seeing eye of our inner nature to join the reality of another person's existence—a person whose inner nature is of the same basic substance as our own. We must dare to embrace our own vulnerability—our own fear of mortality, our own desire for safe anchor in the familiar harbor of home, remembering they have the same deep need for safety and familiarity.

It is essential to understand the importance of reciprocity in this relationship: it cannot be all giving with no getting back. The fire of life inside them can be felt if we get close enough, if we become perceptive and unencumbered enough to feel it. And it will thus kindle our own, as, together, we had felt in the warmth of that room.

The impact and integrity of this kind of interaction has much to do with our intentionality: we must believe relationship is possible, that communication can occur, that the burden of living can be shared, and that moments of connection matter, even if the main content of this time is silence. Importantly, it is a living, breathing silence, made sacred in the sharing.

We come as seekers, as believers, holding one another accountable only to be as fully human as we can be in whatever physical or cognitive state we may be found. If not already apparent, this exercise has as much to do with seeking the core of our own humanity as it does with seeking theirs. Communion is the treasure that awaits. It found us in the session with Janice.

Perhaps Janice had worried she would miss her ride back home to love, familiarity, comfort and belonging. Maybe we had been able temporarily to provide some of those qualities for her. But what had Janice reciprocally provided for us? Something of herself, of her "home?" Had we been, are we, the ones without dementia, looking for home, as well? Had we found it, if for only a few moments, in her eyes?

I suppose one would have to look at the completed collage of everyone's experience of that day to be able to tell for sure. But from my vantage point, I will have to respond in the affirmative.

Because "some things are meant to be."

Beyond the Blue

Art is an appeal against vanishing.[1]
—LYNN CASTEEL HARPER

It has to come from in here.
—JOE

HE WANDERED IN RELUCTANTLY. A sky-blue windbreaker was the first we were to see of him and would be the last (God must have used the same paint for his eyes).

Joe, an eighty-year-old, steel-cast Vietnam veteran, stiffly entered the first art therapy session and sat with crossed arms and pursed lips at the end of a table in the activity room of Caring Days. Two other persons with dementia were present, plus seven students, three researchers, and an art therapist. Two female students assigned to Joe timidly took their places beside him and began the humbling and uncomfortable task of learning how to communicate with someone whose verbal skills were being lost to dementia.

Joe had severe expressive aphasia, the loss of expressive language, though he retained most receptive abilities. Thus, he could understand what was being said but had great difficulty expressing thoughts and feelings through words. His aphasia accompanied three other characteristic

---

1. Harper, *On Vanishing*, 211.

features of Alzheimer's disease: amnesia (memory loss), apraxia (inability to perform familiar tasks), and agnosia (inability to process sensory input).[2]

I sat in the background observing, thinking how much Joe reminded me of my father; both were veterans, about the same size and build, stoic and strong, with the same firm handshake. I wanted to go near and encourage him. To tell him I was proud of him (just for showing up for life), like Dad had always told me. I thought perhaps, at some level, he needed to know.

Dad's favorite color was blue. Sky blue. Like his own eyes. And Joe's.

Witnessing the expression of Dad's personhood through art completely changed my medical practice as I grew empathy, understanding, and hope to inspire anyone on a similar journey. The art had made Dad's spirit sing again, saving both him and his story for all of us.

As BATL emerged from Dad's narrative, our mission came clear: to share his story widely so that others could learn never to stop searching for personhood in those living with dementia or any other disability. I know of no lesson bearing greater importance, not only for care partners and families of persons living with dementia but also for students and healthcare professionals, and for a humanitarian society in general.

"This may be challenging," I whispered to one of the students at the start of the first art therapy session, out of earshot and eyesight of Joe. I wanted to encourage them and to let them know I would be nearby to help.

As our art therapist, Dr. Mildred Dawson-Hardy, explained the first directive, it became apparent that Joe was not going to be making any art. At least, not the art that was called for in the directive. He spent most of the session coaxing his students to draw and cut shapes to place on a white-paper background. Almost no words were understandable, but occasionally, one could make out, "I need to do what I want to do" or "It has to come from in here." And he would put his hand over his heart.

Observing the development of these intergenerational relationships over the past ten years since the program was started has been one of the highlights of my career. Each semester has its relational gems. But none has affected me more profoundly than that of Joe and his two student partners.

We knew very little about Joe. Cared for by family members in a nearby community, he attended Caring Days most days of the week. We later learned that he had once built a home from the ground up, grown and canned his own vegetables, taught line dancing, and greatly looked up

---

2. Described by geriatric psychiatrist and longtime UAB medical school faculty member Dr. Richard Powers as the "four A's of Alzheimer's" (personal communication).

to his father. But right then, Joe was a tough nut to crack, his hard shell impervious to most who tried to engage him. I held out for that almost miraculous transformation I'd seen happen many times before, when the relational phenomenon finally unfolded through a space cleared by mindful listening, compassion, intention, and presence.

Sure enough, gradually, Joe started warming to his new friends. His body language became more open, and he began participating more actively in the art projects. In one very tender exchange after several weeks of art therapy, Joe reached over and touched the hand of one of his student partners, telling her in a halting, stilted voice that she had done a good job with her art. Later that day as they escorted Joe out of the art therapy session, he told his student partners that they were "good people."

The real breakthrough came the day when our musicians, Don Wendorf and Friends, visited an art therapy session, playing and singing familiar songs for the students and their partners, like they do each semester. As the concert progressed, Joe grew more and more joy-filled and happy. By the end of the session, he was dancing with any partner who happened to be nearby. He even came up and placed his arm around me, harmonizing with me on "Amazing Grace." This was a moment of deep connection which I feel at some level will never be forgotten.

We witnessed Joe's spirit breaking through the shackles of dementia that day, singing and dancing its way into all our hearts. Joe's pleasure was infectious. His students were profoundly moved by what happened in that room.

When he left us that day, still radiant with happiness, we did not know that would be the last time we would see Joe's windbreaker-blue eyes and blue soul. Two days later, Joe wandered away from home in the middle of the night. His body was found six weeks afterward in a ravine not far away.

Days passed after we learned he was missing. Then weeks. I am sure his family went through the unimaginable during that time. The students, day-center workers, and I suffered quietly as well. One student, not even one of his two partners, said she had been unable to sleep since Joe's disappearance and could think only of him wandering alone in the cold and rain looking for home with no one to show him. It was heartrending to hear her say this and showed me just how impactful this program and the relationships it fosters are for these young people. Yet, even with the twin memories of Joe's last day with us and his puzzling, tragic disappearance, we had to move on.

Part II: The Stories

When it became apparent that he likely would not return to our program, I met with his students to give them options about how to finish the semester. Either they could stay with Joe, completing his life-legacy book on which they were working with information they already had garnered and impressions they had developed, or we could choose another partner for them with which to work over the remaining weeks. Without hesitation, both said they wanted to stay with Joe, to honor his personhood by creating the best legacy book possible for his family, and simply to express the gratitude they felt for the experience of working with him.

Six weeks later, Joe's body was found.

For the remainder of the semester, Joe's students centered themselves completely on the person they had come to know, interacting together within this personhood during each ninety-minute art therapy session. They reminisced while discussing his unique character traits and the impact he had made on them in a few short weeks. It was as if Joe, in all the deep blue of his selfhood, had sashayed right back into the room.

Finding Joe's remains brought some closure; still, we were haunted by his memory. The students talked often about the relationship they had built with Joe in just five weeks; about how well they knew him. The essence of Joe. His character. Though they had learned so few facts of his story, they seemed to have gleaned the parts that matter most.

Alzheimer's is a thief; only death itself is its equal. But even Alzheimer's can't steal the essence of personhood or the beauty of relationships. Those live on through the power of love. In some essential sense, personhood is relational and is dependent upon those loving interactions that touch the core of who we are. And they develop in the broad and level space of presence: the ground turned holy by the vulnerability and authenticity of persons who choose to enter the reality of another without trying to control it and without losing the integrity of their own personhood. That's what Joe's students did, and I am so proud of them.

I believe personhood is eternally remembered in the mind of God. We can be of the same mind.

As previously mentioned, BATL completes each semester with a celebratory dinner in which the students stand up and say what the experience has meant to them, honoring and validating their partners living with dementia. Though not physically present at this event, Joe was very much with us through the reverence and gratitude expressed as the students shared his story and the transformation it had wrought in their lives: "I'll never forget the time that you told me that my art was good. I'll never forget when you touched my hand. I'll never forget the time that you sang every word to every song alongside Dr. Potts. I'll never forget you saying that I was a good person. I'll never forget you."

In the end, they brought the wanderer back home through a friendship that reached far deeper than fractured phrases and fading memories, stretching clear across the divide of generations and disabilities to a place where we all are one. I wonder if they know they brought themselves back home as well?

There was another presence in the room at the celebration that night. Even if I was the only one who felt it, that made it no less real. Dad's eyes were beaming as big and blue as those of his new friend, Joe.

Art with Mary

"What does art give me? Life! Life!"

—MARY

MARY, A NINETY-FIVE-YEAR-OLD ARTIST living with Alzheimer's disease, nearly sightless from macular degeneration, had one of the most joyful and enlivened spirits imaginable. She quickened everyone around her each time we gathered for art therapy.

Before one particular session, our therapist had talked with me about the challenges of artistically engaging someone with poor eyesight. She had decided to try shaving-cream art because of its use of the tactile sense and thought this might be appealing to Mary.

Mary was always so warm and continuously reached out to all of us in the room. In each session, she started out by telling us how grateful she was to be there, to be included, and about how she feared she would talk too much in the sessions. Also, she spoke about how she couldn't see well. As we delved into this session, she said many times, "Oh, this is just fabulous!"

The therapist started the session with some life-story discussion, which flowed very naturally. Mary told us details about her family, and we reviewed some of the life-story she had shared at the previous session. She told us about her father's cotton farm and about how the cotton used to be used for airplane wings. She mentioned that her husband was a pilot. Then the art activity started. Mary sat at one end of the table, and the students filled the rest of the space (tables were placed in a *T* shape).

Mary then was instructed on how to squirt shaving cream into an aluminum pan, to choose her food coloring, to place drops of her favorite colors in the shaving cream, and then to swirl the colors around in patterns of her choosing with a small wooden stick. Then, she was to blot a piece of watercolor paper into the mix, absorbing the color. At last, she would scrape off the shaving cream, leaving beautiful patterns of color in abstract form.

Mary sat eagerly and affirmed her interest. (Everything about her was affirming.) She had some help from her students, as she admitted she could not see any of the details or colors. She chose red, yellow, and green food coloring, and her students helped her place the colors. The therapist then gave Mary the wooden stick and she stirred in her patterns. The paper was blotted, and then Mary, with help, scraped the cream.

What happened next was miraculous, and I hope always to feel its impact. Since Mary was having trouble seeing the art, the art therapist compassionately and astutely asked the students to tell her what the art meant to them. Then Mary would be in a better position to come up with a title. So, we went around the room, and each one of us told her what the art made us think of, what we felt when looking at it, how it stirred us, etc. When the last person had shared, Mary was asked to title the art based on those comments. Obviously moved, Mary said she thought "Celebration" would be a good name. Tearfully, she then declared, in the same hushed expectancy with which a grandmother might direct a child's attention to a nest of robin hatchlings: "There's something here . . . a new beginning."

She confessed her fears that she would never be able to make art again due to her poor vision, and about how art had meant so much to her in the past. She began to speak of how wonderful her life had been and how grateful and full of joy she was about God's goodness and faithfulness in her life.

She then told all of us, none of whom she could see well enough to make out our faces, how much it meant for her to know that we all were feeling the same thing, that we all were experiencing the power of art to kindle relationship. She said, "I want you all to know it, to really know it, every one of you. How important this is! I am so thankful."

Sharing that the experience was causing memories to flood into her consciousness, Mary spoke about how grateful she was for this. She tenderly recalled her wedding day and how the minister had started a custom that apparently was not being done at that time of having the bride and groom turn and face each other to exchange vows. As she talked about turning to face her husband and exchange the promises, she cried. We felt that the eyes of her imagination were seeing him again, perhaps in the blurred collage of our faces, as the deeply held emotions of one of the most important events of her life replayed themselves. And we realized that, perhaps for the only time in our lives, we were present at the moment when a blind person had regained her sight.

There, in the activity room of an adult daycare center among the young and the old who had come together to create art and make new friends, the curtain of blindness had been lifted, not just for Mary but for all of us; through Mary's newly restored vision, we were enabled to see even into the deepest parts of ourselves.

There are many other details that came out that day. It seemed that the storehouse of the heart had been unlocked. The students were so attuned to what she was saying. Everyone was completely present with each other, and with ourselves, in the moment. Nothing else mattered at that time. And everyone was sharing. Mary went on, "Lord, honey, I didn't know we were gonna have ourselves a prayer meeting today!" Then she added, "God sent you all to me. I just know it." We were experiencing the joy that is possible when one chooses to be present for a person living with dementia.

Much more could be written about the importance of that day. Mary was validated in her current reality in that moment. She was able to create again, and she was so thankful for that. Her spirit and memory were jolted alive by the experience, and she seemed to be imbued with a force that transcended Alzheimer's disease or any other limitation, and it kindled the life in each of us.

Dr. Albert Schweitzer, the great philosopher, theologian, musician, and medical missionary, once said, "The true worth of a man is not to be found in the man himself, but in the colors and textures that come alive in others."[1] Mary's gifts to us were all these many colors to which we had been blind until we knew her. We had come to bring something to her that day. But we received a great blessing. What a privilege to have had that experience!

After that event, one of the students said that in the car on the way home, she and her friends began to open up and share in their own vulnerability, to talk about their heartaches and some of their trials, and to try and meet each other's needs. She said that they all were perplexed at first but then realized it seemed right to do this after Mary's example.

---

1. Schweitzer, "The True Worth . . ."

Art with Mary

They were entering into the vast, expansive warmth of the self shared in relationship with others. They had washed themselves in the healing waters of Mary's joy. They could see.

Thank you, thank you, Mary, for sharing your art with us all.

Amazing Grace with Aretha

I once was lost, but now am found. Was blind, but now I see.
—JOHN NEWTON

ARETHA FRANKLIN WAS A genius. Who could hear her interpretations of African American gospel hymns and spirituals and not be stirred? The gift knew no bounds and was not genre-defined. Her 1998 Grammy Awards rendition of "Nessun Dorma," Luciano Pavarotti's theme song, which she was asked at a moment's notice to sing after the opera star had taken ill, became one of her most revered performances.[1] But for me, her gospel and soul recordings will forever remain in a class by themselves. None is more highly regarded than *Amazing Grace*,[2] her live album recorded at the New Temple Missionary Baptist Church in Los Angeles in 1972, which appears on *Rolling Stone*'s list of "500 Greatest Albums of All Time."[3]

The popular hymn by the same name, "Amazing Grace," ranks among the world's most beloved songs of faith and often crops up in our BATL art therapy sessions. According to a legend popularized by Trinidadian American singer, songwriter, and pastor Wintley Phipps,[4]

---

1. To view a video of Aretha Franklin's performance of "Nessun Dorma" from the 1998 Grammy Awards, see Ignazio Parente, "Aretha Franklin."

2. For more about Aretha Franklin's album *Amazing Grace*, see Wikipedia, s.v. "*Amazing Grace* (Aretha Franklin album)," https://en.wikipedia.org/wiki/Amazing_Grace_%28Aretha_Franklin_album%29.

3. Bernstein et al., "500 Greatest Albums."

4. To watch a video of Wintley Phipps discussing the story of "Amazing Grace," see Gaither Music TV, "Bill & Gloria Gaither."

slave-captain-turned-clergyman John Newton likely heard this melody, which resembles other West African sorrow chants, wafting up from the tormented human cargo of a slave ship and later used it as the framework for the lyrics of poet William Cowper. It is fitting, and even redemptive, that some of the most beloved recordings of the hymn have been made by African American artists like Aretha Franklin.

We found out during art therapy that one of our BATL participants, Martha, an eighty-year-old African American woman with Alzheimer's disease, had been the wife of a late pastor. Memories of church days often filtered forth during art directives, and Martha's students did a fine job of engaging her with nonpressured, open-ended questions about her experiences.

During one particular directive in which greeting cards were made for friends, Martha told us about a cherished childhood friend to whom she would like to compose a card. One of the students showed Martha a card that she herself had made and asked Martha if she had any words of wisdom that she might include on the card to her college friend. Martha replied, "Tell her to try and remember that everything we want is right in front of us; so, simply reach out and take it."

Listening attentively in the background and heeding Martha's advice, I reached out for my cell phone and searched a playlist of songs for Aretha Franklin's version of "Amazing Grace," which we had not yet played during that semester's sessions. That familiar voice again came up out of the earth, settling in those places where deep longings pant to be assuaged.

Almost immediately, Martha's face transfigured, as if she had seen her people, risen imperishable, in the radiant presence of the One who created the grace about which, so often, she had sung. Gently laying down the pen and card she was making for her friend, she slowly turned her face upward unblinkingly, lips moving rhythmically to Cowper's lilting lyrics: "Through many dangers, toils and snares I have already come. Tis' grace hath brought me safe, thus far, and grace will lead me home."[5]

Led by the voices of church folk singing deep down in Aretha's soul, Martha told us of gathering time, of welcoming incoming members while singing, "Oh, How I Love Jesus," of baptisms and communions and prayers and preaching, and of her late husband's pastoral heart and congregational care. She had loved and been grateful for her role as a pastor's wife, she told us as tears trickled down her face and the faces of others who had witnessed

---

5. Doe, *John Newton's Olney Hymns*, 40.

Part II: The Stories

something as ephemeral as a rainbow, yet which promised to pan forth gold from all of our lives.

The voice and the tune and the words had dipped down into the river of Martha's autobiographical memory, and all of us had been immersed. Such is the hidden treasure of long-term memories, especially those which hold meaning and are associated with strong emotions; the neural circuitry in which the memory is stored can be accessed again under the right conditions.[6] The familiar music provided the key; but, as I told the students, the tone had already been set for such a powerful awakening by their building a trusting, validating, supporting atmosphere for Martha and the other participants, a riverside clearing into which the pristine wildness of the human soul could show itself.

"The Lord has promised good to me," she sang. And we believed that she believed it. And we felt that a promise to our friend Martha was surely also a promise to each one of us the day Aretha found Martha and opened up her eyes again, for "as long as life endures."[7]

---

6. Hass-Cohen and Findlay, *Art Therapy*, 57.
7. Doe, *John Newton's Olney Hymns*, 40.

Miss Lola's Purse

Alzheimer's steals so much. Why would I want to participate in the theft?[1]

—TEEPA SNOW

MISS LOLA, A STATELY eighty-five-year-old with Alzheimer's, walked in somewhat hesitantly for the first art therapy session in BATL. She stood taller than most of those in the room, donning a sharp hat and matching purse, which she kept on her shoulder for the entirety of the first three weekly meetings.

After initial introductions, Miss Lola and her students delved into the art therapy directive fairly easily; she seemed increasingly comfortable each week, and the students were more at ease while engaging her. As the rhythm and tone of the sessions started to settle in, a rich cache of life-story material began to show its treasure.

"I'm from Hunter County. Have you heard of that? My Daddy had a store, and Mama sang in the church choir. Daddy had a piano in the store, and we used to sing and dance there. But we didn't tell Mama . . ."

Miss Lola's children were a common topic of discussion. She was obviously quite proud of them. But confusion lurked ever near the surface. One day a few weeks into the semester, she seemed different from the outset. Her eyes were afraid, she was tentative around the students, and there was an undercurrent of angst.

---

1. To learn more about The Alzheimer's Foundation of America's Partners in Care: Supporting Individuals Living with Dementia DVD-Based Training, featuring Teepa Snow and others, see "AFA Partners in Care."

With the students' intention, presence, mindful listening, and validation, she was able to be redirected, and for a time, things got somewhat better. Then she began to get that look again.

"Do you know where I am?"

"Yes, Miss Lola. We are at Caring Days, where we all do art together and get to know each other!"

"Caring Days. Hmm. We are? I'm not very good at art. I'm afraid my children won't know where to find me."

"That's understandable, Miss Lola. But we are here to help. We enjoy spending time with you."

She began to settle again. "I'm very proud. All of them went to school and did so well. They sure do this old heart good."

We knew from things she had said, and by what we had learned from her family and Caring Days staff, that Miss Lola's faith was of central importance to her. But that day, she did something we had not seen her do in past sessions. She began to weave Scripture into her conversation, as per the example below. She seemed to be calling out, speaking her needs, her pain, her confusion, her fears, and then answering herself with passages she had memorized from the Bible. Here is one illustrative exchange between Miss Lola and her students:

"Yes, this old heart is proud. But I am so old now, so very old . . . 'I have been young, and now am old; yet have I not seen the righteous forsaken, nor his seed begging bread.'"

"What was that, Miss Lola?"

"I am old."

"But that makes you wise! We are learning so much from you, Miss Lola. We love hearing stories about your life and family. Would you like to make a collage together? Here, the art therapist has provided us some magazines. Would you like to look through them and see if anything catches your eye?"

"Well, yes, but I don't want to be any trouble to anybody."

"Oh, you're no trouble, Miss Lola. No trouble at all. What would you like to start with?"

"Well, maybe, um. Do you think my children will know where I am? 'The Lord is my shepherd; I shall not want. He maketh me to lie down in green pastures; He leadeth me beside the still waters; He restoreth my soul.'"[2]

---

2. Ps 23:1–3.

Miss Lola's Purse

This pattern continued for most of the session. Then one of the students noticed something the rest of us had missed: *she didn't have her purse with her that day*. Staff went to retrieve it, and shortly after it was given back to her, she began to change. Things started to resemble the past few weeks. And we all (I, especially) could have kicked ourselves for not getting her purse sooner.

After art therapy that day, we processed this teachable moment in some depth. The purse was a portal into familiarity for Miss Lola, probably representing an element or elements of her personhood, helping to secure her identity as confusion circled threateningly. The fact that she was unaware that she was missing her purse poignantly illustrates dementia's effects. But what was our excuse?

We discussed the innate ways humans have of comforting themselves, of leading themselves back to themselves in times of trial or struggle, entering into the formative parts of their stories, and plugging back into the familiar and secure. For many, faith remains an anchor for the self; we believe it was for Miss Lola. And we determined to be more mindful and observant in future sessions.

I believe, though I cannot prove, that there are deep and mysterious comforts available in the inner sanctum of the soul for one who is distressed in dementia's throes. Using the language of faith, grace fills every gap. The only requirements are emptiness and longing.

We should refrain from always saying that someone is "suffering from" Alzheimer's, other dementias, or any condition, for that matter, because such a statement is based on an ego judgment we are making as observers, which may not be the predominant lived experience of the person who has the condition. Surely, we can recognize certain states where pain or distress must be inherent and then surmise that someone may be suffering through them, as we know that we would be as well. But we simply cannot know what the totality of their experience is; though, by honing the power of empathy, we should attempt to try.

In Miss Lola's probable experience of loss and vulnerability (the presence of Alzheimer's disease and the absence of her purse and all it represented), I believe that grace filled the gap with words of Scripture that likely had comforted her and her family many, many times over the decades. And I am thankful that our BATL students were able to help her through being observant, mindful, and supportive.

"I'm afraid my children won't know where to find me."

"We can help, Miss Lola. We all are your children now."

Keep Going!

> If you're going through hell, keep going!
> —WINSTON CHURCHILL

Few of us now living, save combat veterans, law-enforcement personnel, and victims of extreme violence or trauma, have been in situations such as Prime Minister Winston Churchill was referencing in his communications to the British people during World War II. But we all have our struggles and trials, our "hells," and likely can relate to this philosophy on some level.

Sports are not warfare. But the strength of will, determination, utter resolve, and mental/physical toughness required of most athletes in overcoming obstacles to peak performance are occasions for putting the prime minister's advice into practice.

Lifelong involvement in sports as both a champion player and an award-winning coach, and its routine attendant battles with adversity, likely helped to train Coach for the challenge posed by his most formidable opponent: Alzheimer's disease. But we soon learned that he met every challenge with an indomitable will to "keep going."

His physician had said it at one of his follow-up clinic visits, and the phrase apparently fit so well into Coach's game plan that he started using it as a sort of greeting and goodbye for each person with whom he came into contact. "Keep going" was his hello, his goodbye, his advice and challenge for others, as "I'm proud of you" and "I'm strong" had been for my father. I suspect it also became his pledge to his loved ones and his promise to himself. His foundational yes to life's most important questions about his existence.

Keep Going!

Coach's dementia was more advanced than that of most of our participants in that semester of BATL, and this was clearly seen in his interactions with the students, ability to follow instructions outlined in the art therapy directives, and facility with processing abstractions, verbal inputs, etc. He tended to do better with activities that were concrete, and he needed sequential actions outlined so that he could know "where he was going before he got there." More abstract or fluid activities, or ones in which there were no numbered steps, made him anxious and uncomfortable.

Almost all of Coach's artwork contained images of sports, often paired with symbols of love for his wife and other family members and his strong faith. The hand-tracing activity conjured up lines of a football field, a cross standing in some water, and a heart symbolizing love for his wife. "She says I lucked out when I got her, but I say she lucked out with me!" The students had a big laugh, which he seemed to enjoy. He felt right at home with young people, having been a mentor to them for decades, and gave many words of wisdom during our time together.

About midway through the semester, we did shoebox art, a favorite BATL art therapy directive previously described. Coach had trouble with this one at first. Too much chaos and disorganization. Too many factors left up to chance, perhaps. He needed time to devise a strategy. Clearly, we had to have a new game plan.

So, he opened the top of the shoebox, traced lines in the paint drops, positioned the marbles into offense and defense and made the feathers into a goalpost. In short, he constructed a football field and put a pink heart near the fifty-yard line. And his student teammates cheered him on. "Keep going, Coach," they chanted.

"I feel like I have known y'all a long time. Y'all make me feel good," Coach told his students as they walked him back to the main room for lunch.

Gathering information from his family, we found out that the leadership at Coach's church, sensing his struggles and seeking ways to keep him connected to his calling, asked him to help young men in the preparation, process, and aftermath of their baptisms—helping them with their robes, assisting them into the waters of the baptistery, and extending a hand afterward. In this way, Coach was enabled to keep positively influencing young people and giving of himself, his energy, encouragement, and faith, all the while shoring up his selfhood in the act of service to God and community. The church heard and heeded his own call, encouraging him to "keep going" toward heaven when the voice of Alzheimer's was admonishing him to stop in hell.

Part II: The Stories

At the final celebration near the semester's end, when we invited our dementia partners and their families to our celebratory dinner and presented to them their art and life-legacy books, the students stood up and thanked Coach for the experience of getting to know him, of making art together, and of his allowing them to be players on his team.

> The past couple of months have been such an incredible experience . . . From the moment you walked into our art room for the first time, I knew that you were a special person. You immediately lit up the room with your outgoing personality and easygoing way of talking to others. Everyone was always so happy to see you . . . I have learned so much from our times together. From your stories, I have gotten to know what an impactful person that you are and continue to be . . . I am encouraged to try to positively influence others in the same way that you have. You have taught me to never be afraid of trying new things, but most importantly, you have reminded me that every person has a special purpose. I want to find my purpose, as you did in coaching, and be a light to others through that purpose. Thank you so much for being willing and excited to spend time with us through Bringing Art to Life. I consider you to be a very special friend, and I will cherish the time we have had together always!

> I cannot begin to tell you how much of a blessing you have been in my life . . . Each week, you have brought the same vibrant energy to Bringing Art to Life, and you make everyone around you happier because of it. It is very evident that you have lived a life for others, and that is something that I hope I can reciprocate in my life. Through you I have learned to appreciate life a little more. Every week, you tell us that all you are is a coach, but I assure you that you are so much more than that. Every aspect of your life has impacted others for the better, and many people wouldn't be who they are today without you. Thank you for showing me that it is okay to try new things and get out of our comfort zones. You reminded me of this each week, and for that I am forever grateful, because that is where true growth begins . . . Thank you for being true to yourself and opening up with us to create a loving atmosphere so that we could build a relationship together. You are a truly inspiring person.

How does one achieve victory over Alzheimer's? Is this even possible? I would argue that spiritual victory is possible over any adversity; that we become victorious by helping others over the finish line and by allowing

Keep Going!

ourselves to be helped as well. We win by finally believing that keeping on was worth it, that there is truly undying purpose in the will to keep going. When, just past the goalpost, we can begin to make out a face that looks a lot like ours.

With an upraised fist, Coach left the dinner that evening with his signature greeting/goodbye/challenge/promise: "Keep going!"

Thanks to folks like you, Coach, we will.

Part III

Poetry Inspired by BATL

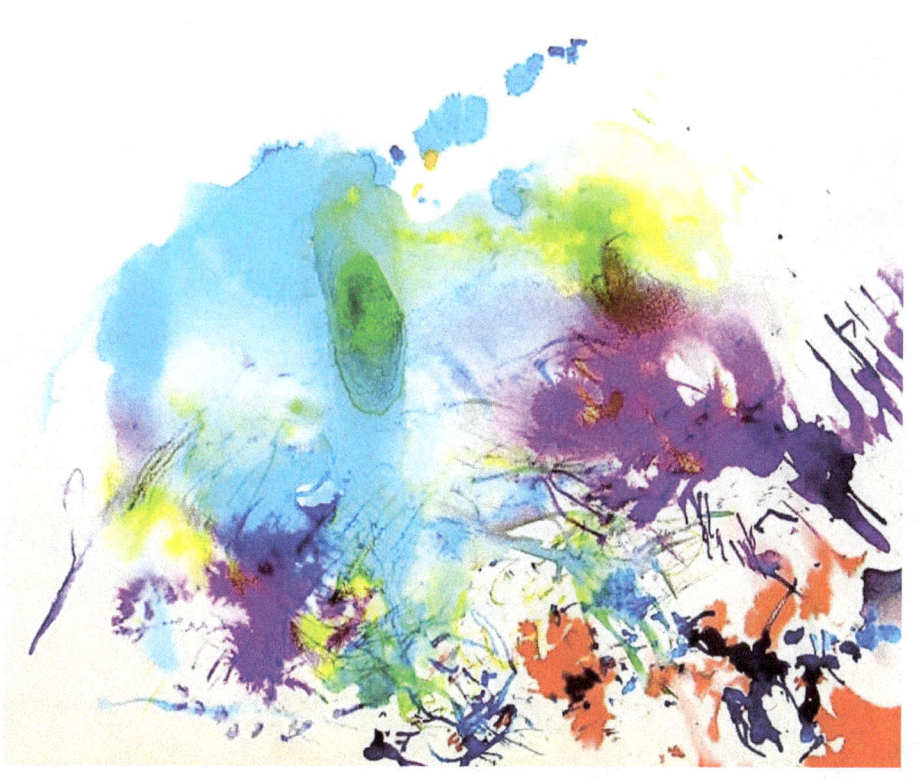

Thoughts on Writing Poetry

> Painting is silent poetry, and poetry is painting that speaks.
> —PLUTARCH

POETRY WRITING HAS CONTINUED to be an essential part of my post-BATL life.[1] I recommend poetry reading and writing to my patients, students, colleagues, and friends, and share poetry that I have written with care partners, in conferences in which I am participating, and on blogs, podcasts, and social media outlets. I am not jockeying for notoriety through published poetry; rather, I hope and believe the deep sharing that is possible through this medium will offer encouragement and hope to others.

In my experience, writing poetry centers one in the present moment and requires intent and mindful focus on words, thoughts, and emotions. The object of one's writing should be something about which one cares deeply if the soul is to be engaged with the words.

During the course of a day, I am struck several times by moments of connection—beautiful scenes, the poignancy of faces, the interplay between light and shadow, the gratitude inherently expressed in the many giftings of life, and the pang of sorrow or pain. I try to record as many of these impressions as I can when they happen. I make a mental note or, if possible, jot down a word or phrase or make a note on my phone that will remind me of why I was moved at the time. Then, I try to come back and write.

---

1. Many of the poems I have written may be found in *The Wooded Path*, my WordPress blog: https://danielcpotts.wordpress.com/.

Part III: Poetry Inspired by BATL

Writing poetry over the period of time since my father's death has made me think poetically. For instance, when a scene captures my attention, often I begin to think of poetic phrases which would describe that scene. Many times, I pair a short verse with a photograph in this way. Learning to think poetically has been a blessing to me over the years and adds a certain grace and exuberance to life—when the conditions are right, on my better days, lifting me above the fray.

My hope in sharing poetry that I have written is to move someone inwardly, not to woo their intellect; to truly and authentically emit the energy of my soul, praying it will connect deeply with others and touch them in ways that are healing, life-giving, and comforting. I hope that something I write would give someone the blessing of diminishing their shame, of causing them to feel gratitude instead of resentment, of creating empathy for someone who may be in danger of being forgotten, or of bringing to light something beautiful that may hitherto have been unseen.

The writing and reading of poetry calls one to a higher plane of life and makes one aspire to something finer, purer, and more authentic; something imbued with truth and integrity and a deep, sacred simplicity that speaks like prayer, a sunset or a river, silence or a song. It helps one to feed those mouths of humility and compassion inside oneself and offers nothing for the rabid throats of selfishness and arrogance. It calls forth one's best.

All of the following poems were directly or indirectly inspired through BATL or the experience with my father's Alzheimer's disease. Often, in my writing, I attempt to speak with empathy in the voices of those living with dementia or care partners. I do this with humility and sensitivity, in hopes that I would not misrepresent the experiences of anyone or serve up any untruth that might look savory to a world waiting with hungry eyes.

Poetry enables the expression of concepts and ideas that are not easily expressed any other way, except perhaps through other forms of art. So that can cause a great sense of resonance in one's inner realms. The poetry is unashamedly spiritual and, in my opinion, must be to do justice to the experience.

The poetry is another way of sharing the stories of all the lives, relationships, and moments that have been a part of BATL since the beginning. I hope that they speak from the very heart of the program.

A Face

In this still and silent moment,
I will hold you. I will hear you. I will keep you.
Confusion. Unfamiliarity. Distortion.
Misunderstanding. Lack of meaning.
Jumbled time. Sunken faces.
Human black holes. The faces.
My face. The mirror. The strangers. The ghosts.
Pounding pulses. Clipped breaths.
Cut-off comforts. Jagged edges. Shame.
Time travels. Lost baggage. Lost home.
Lost people. Little babies. Old women. Mama. Daddy.
Hold me. Help me. Why?
In this still and silent moment,
I will hold you. I will hear you. I will keep you.
I will show you a Face.

A Heart That Knows Your Name

You're the glory in my struggle,
I'm the treasure in your tears.
We will triumph through this trouble
with the life left in our years.
You're the angel in my darkness,
I'm the devil in your dawn.
But a deep peace, like a river,
saves our souls when hope is gone.
There's a Face that's not forgotten.
There's a Person in the pain.
There's a Hand stretched out from Heaven.
There's a Heart that knows your name.
Light a candle in my window
with the fire from your soul.
There'll be green trees in the winter
and a love when blood runs cold.
There's a Face that's not forgotten.
There's a Person in the pain.
There's a Hand stretched out from Heaven.
There's a Heart that knows your name.

A Love-Washed Healing

He'd gone to get groceries
for his mother.
Someone beat him
and left him for dead. But
he hadn't died.
In a coma, he'd remembered
the doctor's grim words
looking down upon his own body.
Later, he'd heard his mother's
whispered prayers and soft singing.
He lived.
It was very hard for him,
but he learned to walk again, to talk.
And his life played out the love songs
he'd heard in another place
like he used to play his saxophone.
He loved.
The students traced his hands on paper.
One partially fisted from paralysis.
One open to the world.
They asked him about himself...
What makes you, you?
What things do you love? Hobbies? Pets?
What's your favorite color?
Together, they helped him draw
parts of himself on the paper.
Here's what happened next.
He drew things he cherished...
His dog, his mother and her flowers,
TV shows and throwing frisbee,

and his saxophone on the tracing
of his crippled hand.
The other hand
he left open and empty.
And all these years later,
knowing he'd let his broken body
be loved back to life again,
we can bring our own crippled parts
for a love-washed healing.

An Elder's Hope

Now I am old, my child.
I bring these years to you.
Know my eyes
until they see from inside you.
Make your pilgrimage
along the furrows of my face.
When you have fallen,
look for truth in the scribbled sand.
Unpocket your hands.
Do not hoard the promise of reaching.
I tell you, life's only dead-end road
leads to the statuary of self.
Turn back from its gleaming stone.
If you see a candle,
find something in your soul
with which to light it.
Learn to find, like I have,
all darkness prescient
with its sleeping gift of dawn.

Bringing Art to Life

Today, I saw something beautiful.
People gathered, happily seeing each other.
There were no expectations.
No regrets. There was only now.
And now was to be lived.
Enjoyed. Together.
Some were young. Some, old.
Who knew which?
They spoke the same joys, fears.
Skipped through the same grass.
Petted the same puppies.
Picked the same flowers.
Loved the same loves.
Spontaneity stole the show.
Gaps were bridged.
Differences honored, accepted.
Personhood affirmed.
Each took a hand.
All came home.

Come On, Join the Choir

Sunrise on another glorious morning.
Somewhere, there's been music all along.
Someone's got a robe for your adorning.
Come on, join the choir. I think you know the song.
Surely, now, you've had your taste of trouble.
Maybe you've grown tired of feeling wrong.
Hungry for a portion, you'll get double.
Come on, join the choir. I think you know the song.
Loneliness has been your habitation.
Even shadows die when light is gone.
At sunrise, there'll be a celebration.
Come on, join the choir. I think you know the song.
Someone wants to see you. Someone knows your name.
Someone wants to sing away the sorrow and the shame.
Listen for the voices. The sound is pure and true.
Someone wants to harmonize with you.
Sunrise on another glorious morning.
Somewhere looks an awful lot like home.
Angels join your anthem of adorning.
Come on, join the choir. And you can lead the song.

Do You Hear Me?

Do you hear me when I say, "I love you?"
Do you know it when I pray your name?
Do you see me beg the sky for answers
as your burning star becomes a flame?
Do you understand my guilt and heartache
for the times I may have been unkind,
when I've held you to some unfair standard,
when your inner light I've failed to find?
If you know these things, I hope you feel me
trying hard to be as strong as you;
striving fast to hear the song you're singing,
to your melody and words, be true.
And I pray an empty place inside you
will be filled with all the love we've known
hand in hand, as now we walk each other
down the old, familiar path toward home.

Hey, Do I Know You?

Hey, do I know you? Have I seen you before?
Just for a moment, I thought, perhaps . . .
Something inside you, peeking out through a door,
made my heart sing once more.
When you reached over, gently taking my hand,
my heart went skipping back home again.
Maybe I saw you in a gray, distant land—
help me to understand.
I see time in a mirror, faded faces of friends.
But relationships never end.
Guess I don't know you. Can you stay where you are?
Let's paint a story to call our own.
Then, when you leave me, I'll be happy you came . . .
somebody knows my name.

Hands upon My Window

Good morning, Lord. How are you?
Is it Monday? Maybe so.
I am thankful that you're near me every day.
I've got a question for you. Something I would like to know.
And I'm grateful that you hear me when I pray.
Lord, it seems the folks who visit
don't come by here anymore.
And, I'm sorry, I don't fully understand.
Are they worried they'll acquire some disease without a cure
if they sit beside my bed and hold my hand?
It may be because I'm hoping
for some unexpected guest,
but I thought, just now, these lonely eyes could see
fingerprints upon my window
where some hands had just been pressed,
and kind faces that were smiling back at me.
Hands upon my window. Faces in my heart.
They help me to get through another day.
Hands upon my window. These faces in my heart . . .
to show me someone hears me when I pray.
And I thought that I heard voices
singing sweetly in my ear,
as the sun was setting warmly in the sky.
And I wanted to sing with them, and I wanted to be near
other singers who are not afraid to die.
Hands upon my window. Faces in my heart.
They help me to get through another day.
Hands upon my window. These faces in my heart . . .
to show me someone hears me when I pray.
And I'm thankful Someone hears me when I pray.

He Can't

"He can't answer those questions.
He can't tell you how he feels.
He stays confused all the time.
He can't tell you what today is
or where he is half the time.
Sometimes, he doesn't even know
who I am, and we've been together
forty years. I have to do most things
for him. He just can't do it anymore.
He used to help around the house.
Not anymore. No help at all.
Can't take care of himself.
He's just not himself anymore."
(Mr. _____ hangs his head,
slowly loses expression in his
down-turned eyes.)
Mr. _____ what do you enjoy?
What makes you happy?
"Spending time with my grandchildren.
Singing. Playing with my little dog.
Tending to my garden."
(Looking up, eyes brighten a bit,
the doused inner fire kindles slightly.)
See, those are things you *can* do.
And those things are most important.
Do those as much as you can.
You don't cease being yourself.
You are you.
You *can*, Mr. _____. You *can*.

Hunter County

My home is in Hunter County.
That's where I was raised.
Do you know where that is?
You see, I'm old.
I finished high school there.
My parents sent me away to college.
All my children finished school.
I used to sing the blues.
Then I got born again.
Excuse me, but . . .
can you tell me where I am?
My children don't know where to find me.
My home is in Hunter County.
That's where I was raised.
Do you know where that is?
I've been born again.

I'll Remember What I Named You

I will hear you in the morning
when you softly call to me.
I will know you in the evening,
though my face you may not see.
I'll be with you in your sorrow,
and my hands will dry your tears
with a promise for tomorrow:
love will conquer all your fears.
Let me be the sweetest mem'ry
that you cannot call to mind.
Let me be the cherished homeland
that you cannot seem to find.
No more wand'ring, lost and lonely
like a wayward ship at sea.
I'm the lighthouse, ever shining.
In your darkness, come to me.
There may come a time, distressing,
when you cannot call my name.
Rest in hope upon this blessing
that is always yours to claim:
I have made you. I have loved you.
And this love will never die.
I'll remember what I named you
in your home beyond the sky.

Life Lesson

We sat together, watching her paint.
Her hands: chorus leaders, loving teachers.
Their movements turning the world.
Turning the pages of her storybook.
Parting the waters so we could go through.
We learned so much of her place and time.
Her inner space. And ours.
The greatest lesson came
as we watched her walk the dark valley,
face upturned, candlelit eyes aglow,
singing her psalms of glory.

Love Holds Us

I'll be the ground you can land on
when you fold your tired wings;
I'll be the rock you can stand on
when your sinking spirit sings.
Let me remember your story:
its pages are part of mine;
show you in all of your glory,
so the world can see you shine.
Don't ever feel that you owe me
for any good deed I do.
If you forget that you know me,
I'll be "Somebody" for you.
When you can't say that you love me
as I quietly take your hand,
I know that God up above me
will help me to understand.
So, let's meet in this moment of living,
You as you, me as me, and be still.
Grace, even unnamed, keeps on giving.
Love holds us, and always will.

Message in a Bottle

On a deep blue day, I will swim to you,
bob like a bottle in the wave-top spray,
so you'll be sure to spot me floating by—
so you'll reach and take the message I've kept
sealed and safe for such a deep-blue-you day,
deep-blue-you-me day:

Even if your day is blue, I'll be there to share it too,
holding tightly to your hand, showing you I understand.
If your head is hanging low, I'll stoop lower so you'll know
a face familiar, kind, and true will always wear a smile for you.
If you can't recall my name, I will love you just the same.
And in the mirror of my heart, reflect, for you, your finest part.

On a deep blue day, I will swim to you.

Poem for an Elder

Today, I choose to see you, dear,
as one in whom the fires of youth
still crackle, as in yesteryear,
yet warmly glow with greater truth.
For that same sprite who played among
a summer's sunlit innocence
still moves with grace in songs unsung
to dance, though falling more than once.
A radiant glow upon the skin
of one too young to know much pain
is lavished on your face again
like sparkling foliage after rain.
The path you chose to grow along
became a space for us to twine;
your spirit's "right" has claimed the "wrong,"
engrafted in the one true Vine.
A quiet strength has been your seal
through toil and triumph, weal and woe,
much as the woodland winds reveal
the depth its forest taproots grow.
The life you live, for all, displays
the water of a stream that flows
within the soul of one who prays
to rest beside the Love it knows.
Of sufferings, you've known your share
and found, inside your one true life,
the weeping wounded everywhere
who seek safe haven in the strife.
From any neighbor standing near
your eyes have dared not turn away,

but listened through their words to hear
what your own broken heart would say.
Thus, beauty you do redefine
in every chapter, every page;
the verses that you underline
are blessings that have come with age.
For such a cherished one as you,
I offer thanks to heaven above,
and pray that God will lead you through
these ever-widening fields of love.

Somebody

If there comes a day when I can't keep from losing
my last mem'ry of the beauty in your face;
when the echoes of your voice seem so confusing
and our home becomes an unfamiliar place,
I am praying that the Lord will smile down on me
and let drops of tender mercy fall like rain,
so my mind can find the words to tell "Somebody"
how their kindness helps to wash away my pain.
And I hope that somewhere deep and safe and certain,
I will not forget the times Somebody shared
the good grace to search the space behind the curtain;
to find the essence of the one for whom they cared . . .
When Somebody saw my failures cast a shadow
over all the sunny mornings I had lost.
When Somebody found me lying in the ghetto
of my wasted dreams and didn't count the cost.
When Somebody said, "I promise I forgive you.
I'll believe in you forever, come what may."
When Somebody said, "I'll take this journey with you,
and together, neither one will lose the way."
And I hope that you will know
in my heart, I need you so.
Though my mem'ries die, my love remains the same.
Will it matter if "Somebody" is your new name?

Someone Is There

Someone is there.

That Someone is not less than
but more than most imagine.

In losing, there may be gains.
We cannot know;
not now.

Here is what we can know:

She can feel and express love.
He has a story and needs to share it.
They are capable of relationships.
They need those relationships.

So do you.
So do I.

Someone to Guide Me

At first, you couldn't see me
through my silence, through my stare,
thinking that dementia meant "nobody's there."

But then, you tried to *be* me
in the moments we could share,
and you found me through your empathizing care.

So, the self that's still inside me,
with its poetry and pain,
found the colors to paint sunshine in the rain.

Now I've got someone to guide me
to my personhood again,
where your loving kindness helps me to remain.

Story Time with Old Folks

I move to silent spaces where the breath stops
and listen to your lines.
The voice of primal life inside you
speaks around and through and under.
Floating in placid expectancy
to where the river slows and widens,
I am found inside the circle of your loves.
Time flows broadly by this island
of reverence and prayer and existence.
All things here are shades of gray.
I see porches on a hill, well-worn rockers,
a steeple rooted in a grove of oaks.
Corn tassels wave the day farewell,
and the called cows come back home.
Barefoot boys take a creek bank by force,
and old ladies weave health into the home place.
Someone sings a song I know from somewhere.
Our people gather at a grave.
Scents of a set table warm and comfort.
Hands with veins of leather reach for mine.
The circle tightens. My soul is loosed.
Love is the only true time traveler.

Take Me to Your Hiding Place

Take me to your hiding place;
there Love's presence fills the space
where lost mem'ries used to be;
is there room inside for me?

There, where fear cannot abide,
I'll be with you, right beside;
faithful to the end I'll be,
'til the lights of home you see.

When confusion clouds your eyes
and you cannot recognize
faces that you've always known,
I'll make sure you're not alone . . .

Let me lead you back again
to the place where we have been
many other times, to see
God still cares for you and me.

The Third Friday in October

On the third Friday in October
as blood-red maple leaves let loose
to dance in the winds of winter
Jimmy told us he's losing his memory
but the Lord has always been good
and he worked for forty-seven years
and he loves his wife and children
and he's glad to be with us today.

This Is Home

Papa looks for home.
He can't seem to find it,
even though he's in it.
We show him pictures,
hoping this will help.
It usually doesn't.
We take him to the old place.
There are vines, rotten boards.
Rusty saw blades.
A bench with no legs.
Distance in his eyes.
No rest. No rest at all.
Always wandering. Searching.
Never finding.
Nothing is sadder than this.
But Papa, dear Daddy,
Look at me. (Lord, still my soul.)
Be with me. Take my hand.
(I'm trusting to the Unseen Hand.)
He leadeth me beside the still waters.
He restoreth my soul.
Let's listen to the crickets.
You are my sunshine.
I never knew you danced so well.
In this quilt (Mama made it),
let me hold you.
Home is here. With me.
Home is in my eyes.
Home is . . .
Home.

Those Girls Came to Visit

Those girls came to visit
on a day she didn't really know,
in a time some talked about
at the edge of cracked clocks
in a crumpled closet corner
of soiled shirts and britches
and the paints they brought
flew in on the flutterings of
winged smiles that floated off
the lips of their butterfly faces
to her own brown blank canvas
and everyone said it was beautiful
and she knew it was beautiful
in a place where few know to look
but they knew and looked inside
and it was good.
So very good.

Was That You?

They asked me why I was going.
"To visit with her," I said.
"But she won't know you're there."
"Perhaps not, but I will," I said.

When I entered,
you were sleeping. Breathing. Still.
I was breathing too.
The air, commingled, held us.
I became still, like you.

Through the window, morning rose.
Birds sang. Spring was present
in flowers and grasses and sunlight.

Listening. Open. Receptive. Aware.
I became no one in the space of the room.

Movement. Reaching. Music. A voice.
Peace. Unity. Warmth. Harmony.
Strangely, the room was an open wound.
And there was water. Cool, clear, clean water.
Pure and holy. And then, the anointing.

The edges of the room drew up
in wholeness; a gathering, an enfolding.

And you sang. Wordlessly, you sang.
To the Presence. To the morning. To me.
A grieving. A prayer. A blessing.

You were sleeping. Breathing. Still.
I left (was it I?), but not the way I had come.

Was that you?

What Are You Planning to Paint?

The world is looking kind of gray.
Sort of faded. You can help.
Your soul has these
beautiful colors in it.
I've seen some
of them come
streaming out
at times like these.
And we can't afford to
miss out on any of your shades.
So, what are you planning to paint today?

When You're Lost

When you're lost inside the shadows
of an unfamiliar place
and you feel the dark around you
for the features of a face,
there's a light that warms and hallows
every God-forsaken space;
so, the darkness won't confound you
as you rest in the embrace
of my Love . . .
of my Love.

There's no fogbank of confusion,
no wilderness of fear
that can hide you from the Spirit's eye
and make you disappear.
For fear is an illusion
that Love has come to clear;
when your mind is in collusion
with those voices that you hear,
I'll speak Love . . .
I'll speak Love.

In the twilight of your memories
I will light a living flame,
and I'll read to you the chapters
of the book that bears your name.

For the person I have named you
is the one you'll always be.
And my boundless grace has claimed you
for a bright eternity
in my Love . . .
in my Love.

Where the Forest Meets the Sky

Part the curtains, dear. I see you.
Put your hand up to the pane.
I am with you, standing out here in the rain.

Please don't worry. My heart hears you
through this window. I'll explain
when the axis of the earth aligns again.

I am praying you'll believe me,
though you can't hear what I say.
It's for your own good that I must stay away.

But the situation grieves me,
and I'm living for the day
I can hold your hand and sing our blues away.

So, just look into my spirit
through the window of my eye . . .
we can see that distant sunset if we try.

Listen closely. Do you hear it?
When I ask if we can fly
in our hearts to where the forest meets the sky?

Wherever She May Go

"Will you be my Valentine?" the lady said to me.
"I don't know where my husband is, or where I seem to be."

Oh yes, I'll be your Valentine; so take this small bouquet
of roses, like the ones I gave you on our wedding day.

For though you cannot call my name or recognize my face,
within love's garden of the heart forever we'll embrace.

So come with this kind stranger you've encountered here by "chance."
Perhaps our soul will play some tune that stirs these feet to dance.

And you'll be swept away again by one who loves you so.
And I'll go with my Valentine wherever she may go.

Yesterday

Yesterday was a big day.
People gathered, something to see.
Someone spoke. There was clarity.
Creativity. Inclusivity.
Folks had pain. Folks had hope.
The young wanted to learn.
To have a new experience.
The old wanted to share.
To make their stories known.
Yesterday was a big day.
Mary gave me a hug.
Gave all of us a hug.
Someone spoke. Mary.
She told all of us she loved us.
Loves us still.
Mary has Alzheimer's.
Mary gave us a hug.
Yesterday.

You Asked Me if I Remember

You asked me if I remember you.
You tell me . . .

I cannot call your name.
I feel that I have seen your face
though I can't be sure.
The lines between maybe me
and maybe you are blurred.
Is this that or that this?
I don't know sometimes.

Yet, I see you now, and I feel comfortable.
Restful. I seem to feel joy here. With you.
I know that someone knows me.
Someone who won't forget. Won't turn away.

I am not ashamed here.
I am not afraid.

Fractured, I feel whole with you.
Needy, I feel I have something to give.
I feel you are open to receiving my gift.

I meet something kind and good.
Something loving and selfless.
I am sure of this somehow.

I feel beautiful. I remember beauty.
And innocence. And laughter.
And running through meadow grass.
And skies of summer, warmly winging.

A new song seems old again.
Dancingly young-old.
Feet touching each other, dusting the floor.
A mysterious making of movement.

With you, the air seems to hold me
safely in rooms where I have wandered.
I can be still here with you.
I don't have to look for words.

But I cannot call your name.
I feel that I have seen your face
though I can't be sure.

You asked me if I remember you.

You tell me . . .

You Chose to Listen

I know you must have been busy.
I'm sure you stay that way.
I suspect there may have been others
who needed you today.
But for me, you made one decision,
a solitary choice,
that changed the color of the world
and gave me back my voice.
My mind's been gripped by confusion,
my memory forgets.
I likely won't recall the names
of faceless silhouettes.
But there's nothing wrong with my feelings,
like sadness, and pain, and joy . . .
there are sheltered spaces in us all
dementia can't destroy.
So, my memory has just recorded,
with the contours of your face,
a true sense of validation,
familiarity, and place . . .
a profound yet nameless knowing,
relational and real,
simply because you cared about
how your actions made me feel.
There, among the busy bodies
brushing by my chair,
you chose to stop and listen for
the soul behind the stare.
When I saw your kind intentions
to truly understand,

it was as if some hidden part of me
went reaching for a hand
that love seemed to be extending through
your presence and your pause
(and I feel the gifts that love extends
it never, yet, withdraws).
In choosing to listen to me, you
did something else, quite rare:
you decided to see what still remains
of the person sitting there,
to regard with respect and compassion,
and perhaps a sense of awe,
the sacred, eternal sanctum of
the suffering self you saw.
In this no one's land of confusion,
you brought a sense of peace,
of trust and vulnerability,
expression and release.
So, my spirit came out of hiding
in the space between us two,
and the air between your eyes and mine
turned the warmest shade of blue
like an iridescent ocean
in backwater of the mind . . .
a place I long to sit beside
but rarely, now, can find.
Please know how deeply thankful that
I am that you stopped by . . .
if I thought about it long enough,
I suspect that I would cry.
But the tears would not be tears of grief
but of gratitude you came,
for your listening has reminded me
Love will not forget my name.

You—Me

You.
You came.
You came and sat.
You came and sat with me.
You came and sat with me when I'd forgotten.
You came and sat with me when I'd forgotten who I was.
You came and sat with me when I'd forgotten.
You came and sat with me.
You came and sat.
You came.
Me.

Part IV

Lessons Learned

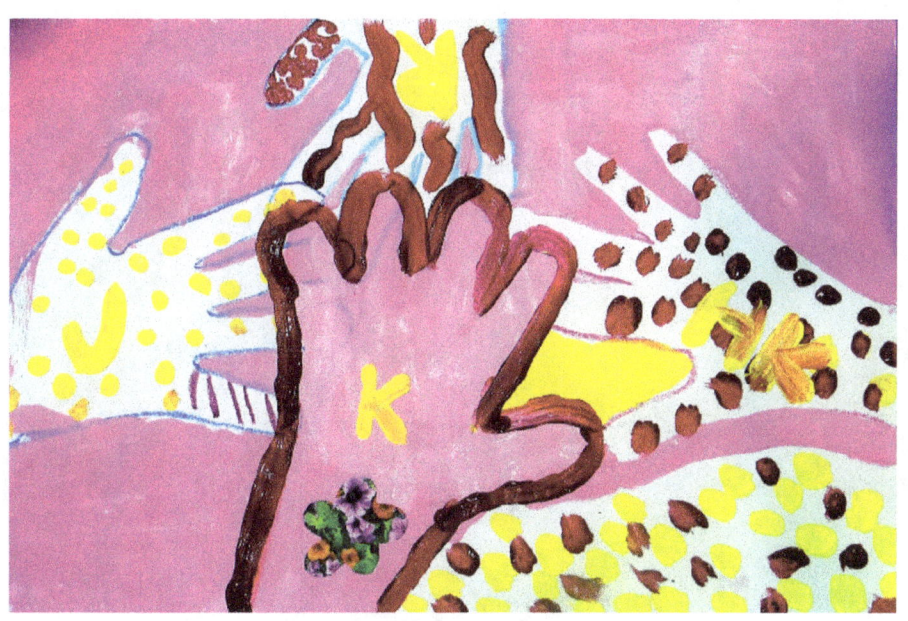

Pillars of Personhood

> I can play a guitar.[1]
> —GLEN CAMPBELL

A Paradigm Honoring Selfhood & Relationships in Dementia Care

- Among those who do not have dementia, one of its most feared consequences is the *presumed loss of personhood*.
- We believe that one of the greatest actual losses in dementia is the *loss of relationship*.
- Loss of relationship is fueled by the stigma of *presumed lost personhood* of those living with dementia ("How can I have a relationship with someone who is no longer there?").
- By faith, we believe personhood is *innate*, *inherent*, and *inviolate*; thus, it is not affected by dementia at the foundational level. Personhood is intrinsically and fundamentally *relational*.
- This belief fosters the provision of *compassionate, dignifying, affirming care* for those living with dementia. Such an environment of care *nurtures meaningful relationships*.

---

1. From the documentary film *Glen Campbell: I'll Be Me* (Keach, *I'll Be Me*).

Part IV: Lessons Learned

- Each individual possesses and retains *self-defining traits* which are enduring, even in the face of dementia.[2]
- Pillars of personhood are those traits that make someone *uniquely who they are*.
- Pillars of personhood may be . . .
  - *Physical*—strength, physical beauty, grace, paralysis, athleticism, etc.
  - *Psychological*—joyful, depressed, narcissistic, kind, gregarious, musical, etc.
  - *Spiritual*—grateful, religious, hopeful, prayerful, serene, giving, talented, etc.
  - *Relational*—family traits, occupation, role in society, values, etc.
- Pillars of personhood are characteristics that would likely be mentioned about a person if they were being honored, eulogized, or remembered among family members and friends.
- For a spouse: "What are the things about your spouse that drew you to him, that caused you to fall in love with her?"
- For a child or friend: "What are the traits that you most admire about your mother, that cause you most to respect her? That you most esteem in your friend? Why do you like to spend time with him?"
- Pillars of personhood do not all have to be traits that are considered good or positive, just authentic or unique.
- Looking for these Pillars and using them as entry portals into the selfhood of persons living with dementia facilitates relationship.
- One may mirror back to another their own Pillars, thus *showing them back to themselves*.
- Pillars may be more easily identified through art, music, and other forms of *creativity*, through *faith* and *spirituality* (in those with that background), through *reminiscence*, through *nature*, in the presence of *children* or *pets*, through the practice of *mindfulness* and *centering* in the present, through shared *laughter* or *tears*, through *imagination* and *storytelling*, and through creating *safe spaces* for *vulnerability, authenticity, validation,* and *presence*.

---

2. These first six bullet points make up the pillars of personhood.

Thirty-One Lessons

Live as if you were to die tomorrow. Learn as if you were to live forever.
—MAHATMA GANDHI

THE FOLLOWING ARE LESSONS that I have learned from persons living with dementia, care partners, and others involved directly or indirectly in BATL. They are taught as part of our educational curriculum in the program. I am thankful for opportunities to be in relationships with, and to learn from, those who are living with dementia.

1. Care partners are curators of another person's museum of life.
2. The innate value and dignity of human beings cannot be stolen by any condition or circumstance. To care with compassion, we must first believe that all people retain an incontrovertible identity.
3. The beauty, vitality, and relational energies inside the very one living with dementia can provide the inspiration for the care partner's journey.
4. We should love and honor persons in their current state, rather than holding them accountable to be what our egos need them to be.
5. Allow persons living with dementia the opportunity to express themselves as completely as they can.
6. Distractions must be minimized during interactions with persons who are living with dementia.

7. We should always look people in the eyes when they are sharing their stories. We should realize that they may be sharing their stories without using words.

8. One's story needs to come out. When words fail, art, in all forms, can be a vehicle for expressing one's story. Expressive arts and opportunities to explore creativity should be made available to everyone who is living with dementia.

9. Nothing stirs the soul more than a feeling of belonging. We must do everything in our power to promote this kind of experience daily in people who are living with dementia.

10. Always try to remember the silent struggles of others, which may lie buried beneath attitudes and behaviors that we don't understand.

11. Rich present-moment experiences open the pages of a person's narrative, bolster identity, and bring a sense of continuity to a person's existence.

12. Laughter is essential. It is the great equalizer. But listening rivals laughter as the best medicine. Listening requires the use of all the senses, not just hearing.

13. We must not take ourselves too seriously. Play is important at any age.

14. It is essential to develop the practice of self-compassion.

15. As care partners, we should act as if our lives are mirrors reflecting only the good and true image of personhood and none of the toxicity of dementia.

16. There is no greater privilege than to help someone find his or her true voice, and no greater crime than to silence it.

17. Culture change cannot occur if the voices of those who are living with dementia are not heard.

18. Don't take it personally if someone living with dementia offends you or hurts your feelings.

19. Empathy is the game changer in creating a culture of compassion in dementia care. Empathy increases when persons allow themselves to have meaningful relationships with those living with dementia. It is especially important to facilitate this process in young people.

20. Though the requirements of care partnerships can sometimes bring out our worst, they also can bring out our best human qualities.
21. Cultivate spiritual intentionality. Get past denial and resentment to acceptance and gratitude. Choose to look for opportunities to love more deeply in each moment of the ongoing care partnership.
22. Reliance upon one's faith and spirituality can provide a deeper meaning to the journey through dementia for everyone involved.
23. Mindfulness is a very important practice to cultivate (for ones living with dementia, care partners, and healthcare providers).
24. Meaningful relationships can be maintained with persons living with dementia even in late stages. Presence is the most important characteristic of these relationships.
25. Brain pathology is not the only determinant of well-being; the relational qualities of one's surroundings play a major role.
26. The strength of the ego's need to retain control often is proportional to the level of denial exhibited by a care partner.
27. It is much better to be kind than to be right. When in doubt, default to kindness. When not in doubt, default to kindness.
28. The need for generativity never goes away. Models of dementia care must address this need.
29. We would do well to remember the things we learn from old people, young people, wounded people, and disabled people.
30. Life is about relationships. That doesn't change if someone has dementia.
31. Personhood, relationships, and empowerment promote living well.

Part V

Final Thoughts

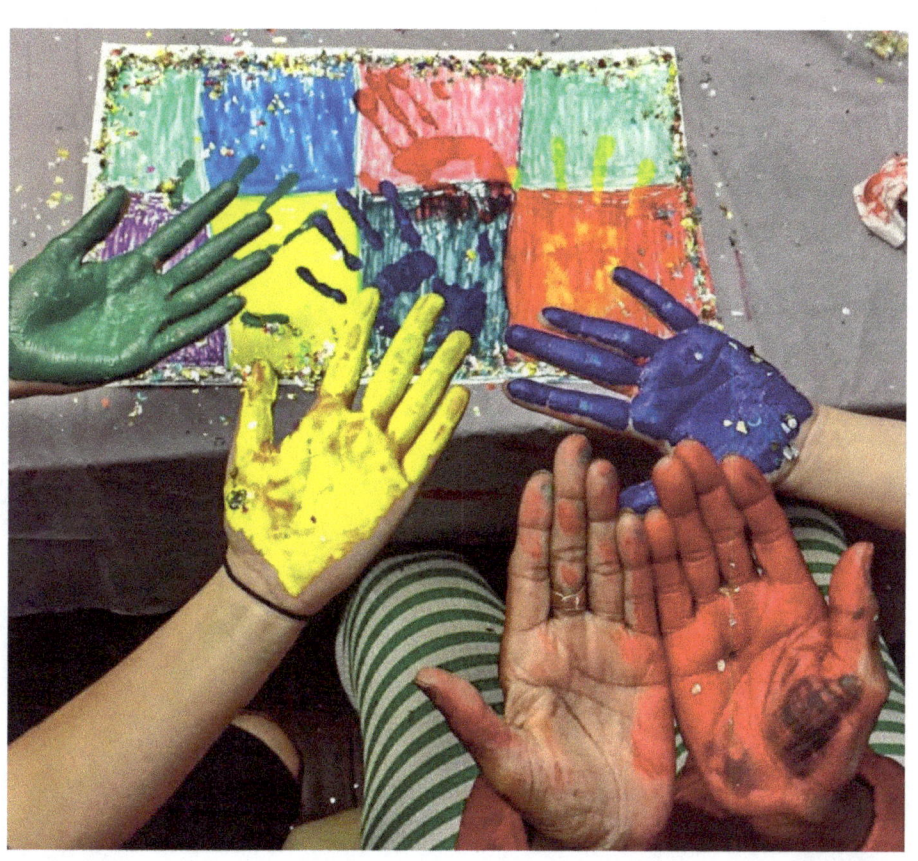

Showing Me Back to Me

> What we have to be is what we are.
> —THOMAS MERTON

BRINGING ART TO LIFE has saved me. Let me try to explain.

In this book's introduction, I discussed writing *The Broken Jar*, a collection of Dad's art and my poetry inspired by that art. My wife came up with the title of the book, a fitting metaphor for Dad. Yet, I had a gnawing premonition that the title would come to describe my life as well.

I felt powerless to do anything about it, locked in the paralyzing gaze of fate. Would this be my mortal wounding? Could my father, and others living with dementia, have felt something similar when confronted with their own terminal brokenness?

Looking into the eyes of fate (reality, death) when you are unable to acknowledge, accept, and grieve over your own powerlessness (a type of death)—indeed, before you have discovered that powerlessness itself must be embraced if life is to be lived with authenticity, vulnerability, purpose, and wholeness—can be a frightening prospect, because you are trying to see with the sightless eyes of the false self.[1] This false self is an artificial persona created early in life to guard one against reexperiencing the trauma of attachment wounds. It is built upon inauthenticity, the invalidation of one's natural emotional responses to the pain or fear of abandonment, and

---

1. Craig, "True Self-False Self," 51–59.

Part V: Final Thoughts

the stifling of healthy self-expression. That's where I had been living. And that's where Alzheimer's was taking aim.

Without exploring too much psychology here, I had built a false identity on attempting to be perfect. By "perfect," I mean striving to conform, as nearly as possible, to the template of the ideal child, student, physician, etc. Feeling that I may have let someone down was the worst possible outcome, especially those who held power over me or those whom I looked up to or respected. When, inevitably, my imperfections showed themselves, I buried them deeply beneath a false façade, denying their presence, and was dishonest with myself about their existence. Thus, a split was rendered in my core, breaching the soul's defenses and laying the groundwork for spiritual illness with the passage of time under conditions of duress. The split, of course, damaged my connection to authentic selfhood, truth, others, the present moment, nature, and the divine.[2]

Throwing myself deeply into work, trying to meet the demands of a young family in a new home, chasing perfection, and attempting to manage the inevitable tensions that occur in intergenerational familial relationships, I burned the candle at both ends without tending to wax and wick. When confronted with the reality of Dad's Alzheimer's disease, my powerlessness over it, and the feeling I was letting him and my mother down by not being able to give the kind of help I longed to give and knew they needed, I sank into a state of panicked helplessness, fear, resentment, depression, self-pity, and shame. Psychological wounds from certain traumas of childhood (all of us have them), unacknowledged and unresolved, fed maladaptive, addictive methods of coping with stress, further contributing to burnout. By the time Dad was entering adult daycare, I was headed into a dark place, feeling bereft and alone.

Then along came Caring Days, George Parker, and the art. Grace to fill the gap. To pick up where powerlessness had come up short. The rescue mission commenced. The inner self would be tended and freed. We would be able to find Dad again, and the parts of ourselves that had been going down with him. They effectively showed Lester back to himself and to us all.

It is alleged that physician, missionary, artist, and visionary Dr. Albert Schweitzer said, "In everyone's life, at some time, our inner fire goes out. It is then burst into flame by an encounter with another human being."[3] Encountering Dad's spirit soaring up through the art lit my fire, and poetry

---

2. Rohr, *Immortal Diamond*, 161.
3. Schweitzer, "In Everyone's Life . . ."

began coming out of me with remarkable fervor, thus making possible the binding up of my soul wounds, a process that would take years and would not proceed in earnest until after my life had hit rock bottom and I had received the help I needed.

Processing later what had happened, I thought of Dad's first painting, the brightly colored hummingbird, wings unfurled to take its flight. I saw the power of the soul, creative selfhood, rising to life transcendent in the shadow of the cruel fate of Alzheimer's, a creature of commingled sorrow and joy, weeping and singing as it flew. I saw this phenomenon drawing others in, sharing its wellspring of energy within an ever-widening circle of influence, claiming for love what had been considered lost to the inevitability of diminishment and death. And I knew that this also described what was happening to me.

Taking this burgeoning enlightenment into my experience with BATL, I began to understand that this was part of a larger framework than just that of education, dementia care, and art making. This was about awakening the inner artist residing in all of us—the creative, knowing, sustaining, nurturing, authentic, ineffable, serene, grounded, true, relational personhood we all possess. The very personhood we claimed existed in all our dementia partners and professed, in our creed, to find and honor through our work with them. BATL was about our dementia partners, their care partners, and our students, about you and about me, and about the broader community. And I knew this discovery could save us all.

The program, then, is about finding the art of transcendent, authentic, creative, relational selfhood, first in others, then in ourselves, letting it change our lives in empathetic, generative, compassionate, and loving ways and telling the world the stories of our discoveries as we each add our unique contribution to a culture of compassion.

Each day in BATL is a day of growth for me. Through relationships with persons living with dementia, I have learned more than I could have imagined. Their courage, resiliency, adaptability, strength, friendship, and authenticity are ever inspiring.

Care partners also have been my teachers. The call to care partnership is a call to the highest human aspirations, a call to others-centered living by the dictates of love. The raw truth is that its demands can bring out both our best and our worst qualities. But I have learned more about forgiveness from care partners than from almost anyone else. And this extends to forgiveness offered not only to others but also to oneself.

Part V: Final Thoughts

Students in BATL have also been my instructors and mentors as well. I have yet to see a student who has not experienced growth and some degree of transformation through relationships with their partners living with dementia. They themselves have shown such courage and maturity in embarking on this journey of uncertainty, and have demonstrated heartwarming empathy and compassion. I have seen this change their relationships even among their peers and have heard many stories from them about how they have become more vulnerable, more accepting of others, and more willing to share their own authentic stories of struggle and triumph.

Countless times, I have been brought to the point of tears in reading student journals about their experiences in BATL and about how willingness to enter into a relationship with someone who is different from them—someone living with a disabling disease like dementia who may be much older than they—has unified their view of humanity, helped them gain self-knowledge, and enabled them to cultivate a mindful approach to life, with a present-centeredness that aids them in coping with the pressures and stresses of their education. This is the part I could not have predicted when we first had the idea to start the program, thinking of it only as a means of helping persons who are living with dementia and their care partners.

I suppose you could say that all of us in the program have been about the task of bringing art to life in each other's lives. Of showing each other back to ourselves. And I can't think of anything more worthwhile to be doing.

Mine is one life that has been saved in the process. That's why I am able to write this book.

Postlude

No day shall erase you from the memory of time.[1]

—VIRGIL

THESE ARE THE STORIES. Their stories. *Our* stories. All of them, threads for a quilt. We have committed to preserving them, to weaving them deftly into the fabric of our days. Thus, bringing art to life.

I remember hearing this tale, though I can't recall the source. A wise and aged teacher lay bereft, bemoaning to an elder former pupil how his life and teachings had been in vain, how there would be no one to remember his story. The pupil responded reassuringly:

> My good master, take heart in your repose. Your life and teachings have made a great impact on many. Recently, I witnessed a pupil of one of my former students living out elements of your story in his own narrative. I was struck by this vision of what must have been you in youthful age. Truly, to have lived is to know that one's story is being told through other lives. Nothing has been in vain.[2]

Writing these words, I sit amidst the social isolation and restrictions of the COVID-19 pandemic of 2020/21. Caring Days, the adult daycare center that my father attended and in which most of the stories relayed in this book have taken place, of necessity was closed for months. BATL was

---

1. This quote from Virgil is inscribed on the 9/11 Memorial in New York City.
2. I have heard this story told in several different ways by various teachers and mentors.

Part V: Final Thoughts

placed on hold for a while as we modified for social distancing and now has resumed in a new virtual paradigm that has been impactful and effective, per testimonials we have received.

During this time, I have grieved for persons living with dementia and their care partners as they have struggled without the benefit of adult daycare and respite programs which had provided such a boost to their well-being. I have grieved for the staff of these programs, whose caring hearts, I imagine, have been pained. I have grieved for residents of long-term care facilities and their families stuck in isolation. I have grieved for those who have lost loved ones and who could not be with them in the final moments.

But I applaud the innovative ways facilities and organizations have continued to provide for their people through distanced sing-alongs, drive-bys, etc., and I know the resiliency, flexibility, energy, and compassion that characterize dementia-care organizations and care partners. Thus, the colors of hope still fly high above the COVID-19-built ramparts of isolation.

Pandemic notwithstanding, I know that nothing can take away the impact we have on each other through relationships that get to the core of our humanity, to the shared story of what it means to exist in the terror and wonder of our days. And the epic nature of this existence builds a narrative much more compelling than the dire headlines of these times or any others. Indeed, art brings itself to life from the refuse and riches of our lives. Life transcends death by becoming death and yet still living.

The fact is that when opposing entities or situations encounter each other—when it seems there is no way past the stalemate but for each to collapse upon itself or turn to fight or devour the other—often a third thing is born of seeming impossibility, a thing which does not deny but accepts and transcends; which does not fear but loves and claims; which does not fold or fight but embraces and grows; which does not bury itself but sings itself to the skies—art is another name for this third thing.

Art is born from these threads of life and death—shades of joy and sorrow, lyrics of comfort and pain, movements of laughter and weeping, melodies of peace and anxiety, stories of triumph and tragedy—reimagined. Art comes from the courage to see the faces of reality and to sit silently and lovingly between them, thus bringing them together. Art is a major component of the grace that fills the gaps. And all of us in BATL have found ourselves in those gaps. Oh, what a privilege to be there!

In advanced Alzheimer's, when my father no longer could speak, I heard his story sharing itself poetically in my voice through colors his art

Postlude

had awakened. I tried to listen, then penned these words for him (perhaps he painted them for me) . . .

> Remember who you are, my child,
> who you were born to be.
> Let love be law in mind and heart;
> let life be charity.
> If bandaged, begging hands assail
> your palisades of calm,
> let labor bring tranquility;
> let healing be its balm.
> When death itself so stealthily
> advances through your days,
> let quiet faith be your resolve;
> let living be your praise.
> Then, when my spirit and my flesh
> unknit and I am gone,
> within your heart, the finest part
> of me continues on.[3]

And I will count on the fact that it continues. I cherish that thought. I resolve that no matter what happens, it will continue on.

So, to our dear friends from Bringing Art to Life, wherever you may be, and to all whom we love and esteem, we make you this promise: we will strive always to honor your art and your stories through the living of good lives in ways that your lives, too, were good. There may come times of unawareness when some promises are forgotten. Rest assured that in mysterious ways, the truth of your lives will continue to speak when we are present—to ourselves, to others, and to God.

And someone, somewhere, may come to know you, may come to love your art and your story, though they cannot call your name. Perhaps they will smile while painting your face on a sunset, bringing art to life.

Finally, I make this pledge to all those who are living with dementia and to all those who aren't: I promise to look for the place inside you that keeps dancing when the music ends, that paints when it seems that life has lost its colors, that laughs in the center of the storm; the place where a silent yes answers every no that is uttered, those hallowed halls of selfhood where the gala showing is you, where the sound of your name echoes forever in the hidden chambers of time. Through this portal, I will be able to enter

---

3. Potts, *Heart That Knows*, 84.

Part V: Final Thoughts

into the gallery of myself. You will be there too, and we will be very much alive.

Reader, I invite you to make this pledge with me.

If you or your organization are interested in Bringing Art to Life, please contact us at info@cognitivedynamics.org.

—Daniel C. Potts, MD, FAAN
Tuscaloosa, Alabama, September 6, 2021
(my parents' sixty-second wedding anniversary)

About the Author

DANIEL C. POTTS, MD, is a Fellow of the American Academy of Neurology (FAAN) and a neurologist, author, educator, and champion of those living with Alzheimer's disease and other dementias and their care partners. Selected by the American Academy of Neurology as the 2008 Donald M. Palatucci Advocate of the Year, he also has been designated an Architect of Change by Maria Shriver. In 2016, he was chosen by the University of Alabama Medical Alumni Association as a recipient of the Martha Myers Role Model Award, which honors physician alumni whose lives epitomize the ideal of service to their communities. And he was given the 2020 Physician of the Year Award by the Association of the US Army, West Alabama Chapter. Inspired by his father's transformation from sawmiller to watercolor artist in the throes of dementia through person-centered care and the expressive arts, Dr. Potts seeks to make these therapies more widely available through his foundation, Cognitive Dynamics. Additionally, he is passionate about promoting self-preservation and dignity for all persons with cognitive impairment. He lives with his wife, Ellen; daughters, Julie and Maria; and miniature Dachshund, Heidi, in Tuscaloosa, Alabama.

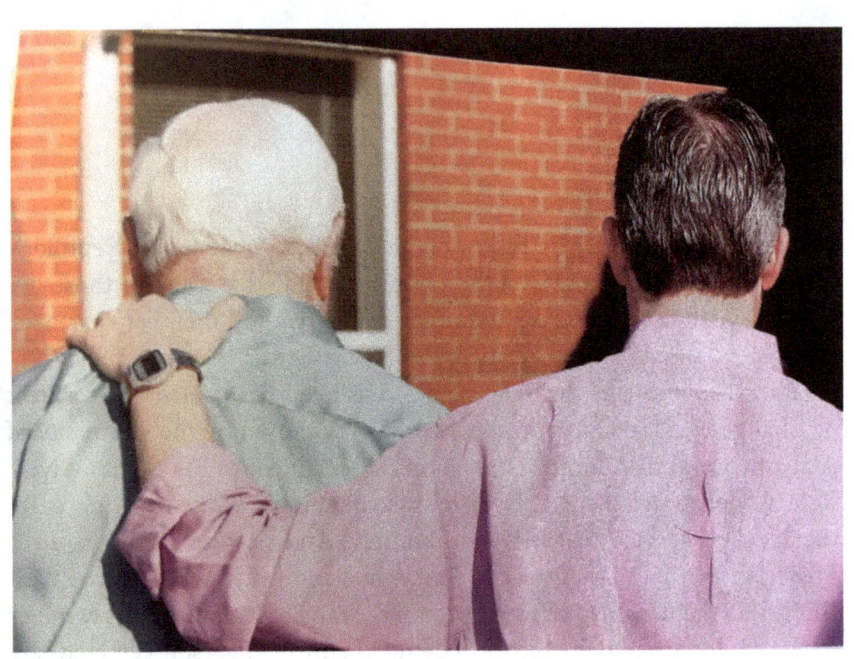

Bibliography

"AFA Partners in Care." https://alzfdn.org/partners-in-care/.
Allen, Rebecca S., and Keisha Carden. "Bridging the Past and the Future: Why Age Matters in Behavioral Health Training." Symposium presented at the Annual Meeting of the Gerontological Society of America, Philadelphia, June 2020.
"Alzheimer's Study Quilt Project." https://www.adcs.org/alzheimers-study-quilt-project/.
Angelou, Maya. *I Know Why the Caged Bird Sings*. New York: Random House, 2009.
Balas, J., and Neelum Aggarwal. "Optimizing a Dementia-Focused Virtual Reality-Based Training Curriculum for Certified Nursing Assistants on the Front Lines of the COVID-19 Pandemic." Poster Presentation at the American Medical Association Meeting, Chicago, April 2021.
Basting, Anne. *Creative Care: A Revolutionary Approach to Dementia and Elder Care*. New York: HarperOne, 2021.
Bernstein, Jonathan, et al. "The 500 Greatest Albums of All Time." *Rolling Stone*, September 22, 2020. https://www.rollingstone.com/music/music-lists/best-albums-of-all-time-1062063/rufus-chaka-khan-ask-rufus-1062734/.
Blandin, Kesstan, and Renee Pepin. "Dementia Grief: A Theoretical Model of a Unique Grief Experience." *Dementia (London)* 16 (2017) 67–78.
Borrie, Cathie. *The Long Hello: Memory, My Mother, and Me*. New York: Arcade, 2016.
Buber, Martin. *I and Thou*. New York: Simon & Schuster, 1971.
"Caregiving." https://thewomensalzheimersmovement.org/caregiving/.
CognitiveDynamics1. "Bringing Art to Life in Beverly Hills." June 29, 2013. YouTube video, 4:24. https://www.youtube.com/watch?v=DTDOkS1unm8.
CognitiveDynamics1. "Do You Know Me Now?" March 9, 2019. YouTube video, 27:35. https://www.youtube.com/watch?v=ivyNozOfz74.
CognitiveDynamics1. "Personhood in Dementia." October 25, 2015. YouTube video, 39:58. https://www.youtube.com/watch?v=7CVt3WqUtg4.
Coles, Robert. *The Erik Erikson Reader*. New York: W. W. Norton & Company, 2001.
Craig, Robert. "True Self-False Self: The Educational Theory of Thomas Merton." *Journal of Thought* 29 (1994) 51–59.
Doe, Charles J., comp. *John Newton's Olney Hymns*. Minneapolis: Curiosmith, 2011.
Ellena, Eric, and Berna Huebner, dirs. *I Remember Better When I Paint*. 54 min. French Connection Films and Hilgos Foundation, 2009.

Bibliography

Everman, Lynda, and Don Wendorf, eds. *Dementia-Friendly Worship: A Multifaith Handbook for Chaplains, Clergy, and Faith Communities.* London: Jessica Kingsley, 2019.

———. *Stolen Memories: An Alzheimer's Stole Ministry and Tallit Initiative.* Eugene, OR: Resource, 2019.

"Excellence in Care Dementia Program of Distinction Care Settings." https://alzfdn.org/excellence-in-care-dementia-program-of-distinction-care-settings/.

Feil, Naomi. *The Validation Breakthrough.* 3rd ed. Baltimore: Health Professions Press, 2012.

Fox, Matthew. *Meister Eckhart: A Mystic Warrior for Our Times.* Novato, CA: New World Library, 2014.

Gaither Music TV. "Bill & Gloria Gaither—Amazing Grace ft. Wintley Phipps (Live)." April 6, 2012. YouTube video, 8:35. https://www.youtube.com/watch?v=qNuQbJst4Lk.

Golden, Marita, ed. *Us Against Alzheimer's: Stories of Family, Love and Faith.* New York: Arcade, 2019.

Harper, Lynn C. *On Vanishing: Mortality, Dementia, and What It Means to Disappear.* New York: Catapult, 2020.

Hass-Cohen, Noah, and Joanna Findlay. *Art Therapy and the Neuroscience of Relationships, Creativity and Resiliency.* New York: W. W. Norton & Company, 2015.

Ignazio Parente. "Aretha Franklin 'Nessun Dorma' Live[HD] (Grammy Awards)." September 26, 2019. YouTube video, 4:46. https://www.youtube.com/watch?v=uHb75oTHOV4.

Ivey, Keisha D., et al. "The Effects of an Intergenerational Service-Learning Experience on Ageist Attitudes." Poster presentation at the IAGG World Conference of Gerontology and Geriatrics, San Francisco, November 2017.

Keach, James, dir. *Glen Campbell: I'll Be Me.* 116 min. Area23a and Virgil Films, 2014.

McLeod, Saul. "Erik Erikson's Stages of Psychosocial Development." https://www.simplypsychology.org/Erik-Erikson.html.

Miranda, Lin-Manuel, and Jeremy McCarter. *Hamilton the Revolution.* New York: Grand Central, 2016.

Morgan, Richard, and Daniel Potts. *Treasure for Alzheimer's: Reflecting on Experiences with the Art of Lester E. Potts, Jr.* Scotts Valley, CA: CreateSpace, 2015.

Morgan, Richard, and Jane Thibault. *No Act of Love Is Ever Wasted.* Nashville: Upper Room, 2009.

O'Neal, David, ed. *Meister Eckhart: From Whom God Hid Nothing.* Boston: New Seeds, 2012.

"Our Story." https://www.alz.org/about/our_story.

"Palatucci Advocacy Leadership." https://www.aan.com/education/palatucci-advocacy-leadership-forum.

Penn, Arthur, dir. *The Miracle Worker.* 106 min. United Artists, 1962.

Pinquart, Martin, and Sylvia Sorensen. "Differences between Caregivers and Noncaregivers in Psychological Health and Physical Health: A Meta-Analysis. *Psychology and Aging* 18 (2003) 250–67.

Potts, Daniel C. *The Broken Jar.* Tuscaloosa, AL: Wordway, 2006.

Bibliography

———. *A Heart That Knows Your Name: Poetry Inspired by Persons Living with Dementia and Care Partners.* Tuscaloosa, AL: Cognitive Dynamics Foundation, 2019.

Potts, Ellen, and Daniel. *A Pocket Guide for the Alzheimer's Care Giver.* Tuscaloosa, AL. Dementia Dynamics, 2011.

"Rebecca S. Allen, PhD, ABPP." https://rsallen.people.ua.edu/.

Reel, Candice D., et al. "Bringing Art to Life: Social and Activity Engagement through Art in Persons Living with Dementia." *Clinical Gerontolology* 8 (2021) 1–11.

Rodin, Auguste. "The Main Thing . . ." https://www.goodreads.com/quotes/39936-the-main-thing-is-to-be-moved-to-love-to.

Rohr, Richard. *Immortal Diamond: The Search for Our True Self.* Hoboken, NJ: John Wiley & Sons, 2013.

———. *Just This: Prompts and Practices for Contemplation.* Albuquerque, NM: Center for Action & Contemplation, 2017.

———. *The Naked Now.* New York: The Crossroad, 2009.

Rossato-Bennett, Michael. *Alive Inside: A Story of Music and Memory.* 78 min. Projector Media, 2014.

Schweitzer, Albert. "In Everyone's Life . . ." https://www.goodreads.com/quotes/12028-in-everyone-s-life-at-some-time-our-inner-fire-goes.

———. "The True Worth . . ." https://breakthroughquotes.com/quote/albert-schweitzer/the-true-worth-is-not-to-be-found-in-man-himself-but-in-the-colors-and-texture-that-come-alive-in-others/.

Shaw, Carrie, et al. "Enhancing Dementia Care and Building Empathy through the Integration of Virtual Reality Technology and Art Therapy." Poster presentation at the Alzheimer's Association International Conference, Chicago, October 2018.

St. Claire, Kassia. *The Secret Lives of Color.* New York: Penguin, 2017.

Swinton, John. *Dementia: Living in the Memories of God.* Grand Rapids: Eerdmans, 2012.

"Thin Places, Holy Spaces: Where Do You Encounter God?" *A Sacred Journey: Practicing Pilgrimage at Home and Abroad* (blog). https://www.asacredjourney.net/thin-places/.

Thoreau, Henry David. "It's Not What . . ." https://www.brainyquote.com/quotes/henry_david_thoreau_106041.

UAB Magazine. "Painting in Twilight: An Artist's Escape from Alzheimer's." May 20, 2009. YouTube video, 7:45. https://www.youtube.com/watch?v=I_Te-s6M4qc.

Walker, Alice. *The Color Purple.* New York: Harcourt, 1982.

Wendorf, Don. *Caregiver Carols: A Musical, Emotional Memoir.* Scotts Valley, CA: CreateSpace, 2014.

Van Dyke, Henry. *The Poems of Henry Van Dyke.* 2nd ed. Amsterdam: Fredonia, 2004.

Vaillancourt, Laura. "Pillars of Personhood with Daniel C. Potts, MD, FAAN." August 9, 2021. Episode 17 of *Life on Repeat: A Dementia Caregiver Podcast.* https://www.lifeonrepeatpodcast.com/episode/pillars-of-personhood.

www.ingramcontent.com/pod-product-compliance
Lightning Source LLC
Chambersburg PA
CBHW071504150426
43191CB00009B/1406